Managing Your Practice Finances

Strategies for Budgeting, Funding, and Business Planning

APA PRACTITIONER'S TOOLBOX SERIES

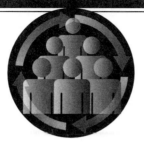

NATIONAL UNIVERSITY
LIBRARY   SACRAMENTO

Managing Your Practice Finances

Strategies for Budgeting, Funding, and Business Planning

American Psychological Association Practice Directorate
with
Coopers & Lybrand, L.L.P.

AMERICAN PSYCHOLOGICAL ASSOCIATION
Washington, DC

A Cautionary Note:

This manual was written to serve both as a reference and as a tool to help providers practice more efficiently in a changing, demanding marketplace. The information contained herein is accurate and complete to the best of our knowledge. However, *Managing Your Practice Finances: Strategies for Budgeting, Funding, and Business Planning* should be read with the understanding that it is meant as a supplement, not a substitute, for sound legal, accounting, business, or other professional consulting services. When such services are required, the assistance of a competent professional should be sought.

Copyright © 1996 by the American Psychological Association.
All rights reserved. Except as permitted under the United States Copyright Act of 1976, no part of this publication may be reproduced or distributed in any form or by any means, or stored in a database or retrieval system, without the prior written permission of the publisher.

Published by
American Psychological Association
750 First Street, NE
Washington, DC 20002

Copies may be ordered from
APA Order Department
P.O. Box 2710
Hyattsville, MD 20784

Composition and Printing: National Academy Press, Washington, DC
Cover Designer: Leigh Coriale

Library of Congress Cataloging-in-Publication Data
Managing your practice finances : strategies for budgeting, funding, and business
    planning / American Psychological Association Directorate with Coopers &
    Lybrand.
        p.   cm. — (APA practitioners toolbox series)
    Includes bibliographical references.
    ISBN 1-55798-361-5 (alk. paper)
    1. Mental health services—Management.   I. American Psychological Associa-
tion. Practice Directorate. II. Coopers & Lybrand.   III. Series
    RC790.75.M36   1996
    616.89′0068′1—dc20   95-52586
                                                                             CIP

British Library Cataloguing-In-Publication Data
A CIP record is available from the British Library

Printed in the United States of America
First Edition

Contents

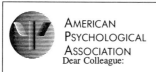

AMERICAN
PSYCHOLOGICAL
ASSOCIATION
Dear Colleague:

The American Psychological Association Practice Directorate is pleased to offer <u>Managing Your Practice Finances: Strategies for Budgeting, Funding, and Business Planning</u> as one component the "APA Practitioner's Toolbox Series" written in conjunction with Coopers & Lybrand, L.L.P. This series of books is designed to help the practicing psychologist build a successful practice in an environment which requires attention to an increasingly complex approach to healthcare while maintaining the quality of services for which psychology has become known. This particular book is intended to help practitioners grapple with the many financial issues related to providing services in today's healthcare climate.

Traditionally, the provision of healthcare was based on a fee-for-service indemnity model of reimbursement. The provider and patient focused almost exclusively on the clinical aspects of care and paid little attention to the financial aspects. As long as the care being provided fell within the general parameters of a patient's insurance policy, the third-party payer insurance company typically paid for the services minus any beneficiary co-payment. The result of this traditional system was little if any incentive for either the provider or patient to be concerned with the financial aspects of care.

Today, by contrast, considerable emphasis is being placed on financial considerations, owing largely to the excessively high costs of healthcare resulting from the traditional indemnity model of reimbursement. All parties involved, including providers, must now attend to the financial and economic aspects of providing health services. In fact, to the extent that providers as a group do not concern themselves with the financial issues related to care, experience suggests intensified efforts on the part of payers and the managed care industry to step in and demand financial accountability. Providers in today's healthcare system, therefore, must integrate financial concerns with clinical concerns in order both to maintain fiscal accountability and to maximize their autonomy from outside parties.

Whether practicing as a solo provider, a partner in a group practice, or as part of an integrated delivery system, attention to the clinical aspects of healthcare must be balanced with a corresponding focus on the financial aspects. Good business, including sound financial planning and management, have become as important to psychology practice as evaluation, diagnosis, and treatment.

Sincerely,

Russ Newman, Ph.D., J.D.
Executive Director for Professional Practice

750 First Street, NE
Washington, DC 20002-4242
(202) 336-5913
(202) 336-5797 Fax
(202) 336-6123 TDD

Russ Newman, Ph.D., J.D.
Executive Director
Practice Directorate

Preface

Financing a psychological practice is an important task. Capital (money) is an enabling factor that allows psychological practices to begin and grow. Providers need funds to lease or purchase office space and working capital to pay monthly bills as patient revenues begin. There are several financial issues that providers should be familiar with: budgeting, funding sources, funding procedures, and business plans.

The business issues described in this guidebook may appear to be overwhelming, and some providers will understand the concepts more easily than others. A practitioner need not try to accomplish all the tasks described here without help. Assistance with financial matters can be obtained from various sources: accountants, consultants, local college or university small business development centers, and the Small Business Administration, among others.

The concepts and procedures involved in budgeting also are discussed here, especially for practices just starting, those in financial trouble, and those wanting to expand. The budgeting process can assist decision making and achievement of goals. Funding requirements determined in the budgeting process drive the personnel and technical resources that allow a practice to expand its ability to provide patient care.

Also discussed are the various types of financing that are available and the purpose each serves. The selection process used to evaluate sources of capital is reviewed, as well as the process lenders use when evaluating loan applicants. Finally, the book outlines the importance of a practice's business plan to the financing process.

HOW TO USE THIS GUIDEBOOK

There are several steps involved in financing a psychological practice. Many people may think of financing as going to a bank to take out a loan.

In reality going to the bank is one of the final steps in the process. This guidebook begins by discussing the financial needs of a behavioral health practice, explores opportunities for capital as the practice wishes to make capital purchases or merge with other practices, and discusses and outlines the need for a business plan.

Chapter 1 reviews planning and budgeting for operations. This chapter discusses setting goals and objectives for the practice, followed by a discussion of the development of a comprehensive budget. It then examines the concepts of profit plans, cash budgets, and balance sheets. Finally, the chapter reviews the concept of flexible budgeting and tools that a practice can use to analyze differences between a budget and actual experience.

Chapter 2 explores the various types of financing that are available. After undergoing the planning and budgeting process, the next step for a practice in the financing process is to select the type of financing that best meets its objectives. Each type of financing differs in cost, flexibility, and restraints. Financing is classified as either debt (which must be repaid) or equity (which results in the exchange of some portion of practice ownership to the lender).

Chapter 3 focuses on lenders, including banks, leasing companies, thrift institutions, life insurance companies, and venture capitalists. This chapter reviews the process that a practice undergoes in selecting a financing source. Finally, there is a discussion of the evaluation process used by lenders.

The final chapter outlines the development of a business plan. Business plans are often key to obtaining financing. The chapter details the typical elements of a plan: a statement of objectives, organization, market data, description of services, and financial statements. Last, it examines the business plan as a practice tool and provides a short overview of personal financial statements.

Acknowledgments

This book was written by Tina E. Kind, MBA, of Coopers & Lybrand LLP. Ms Kind is a consultant with Coopers & Lybrand's Health and Welfare Practice in Atlanta.

The following individuals from both the American Psychological Association and Coopers & Lybrand were instrumental in providing editorial assistance toward the successful completion of this work:

American Psychological Association
Russ Newman, PhD, JD
C. Henry Engleka
Chris Vein
Craig Olswang
Garth Huston

Coopers & Lybrand, LLP
Ronald A. Finch, EdD
Wanda Bishop
Alfred E. Schellhorn, MBA

1

Planning and Budgeting for Operations

THIS CHAPTER DETAILS *financial budgeting for a psychological practice. The techniques discussed here serve as the basis for analyzing funding requirements and obtaining financing. Along with a short discussion of setting goals and objectives, the chapter covers preparation of a comprehensive budget and the concepts of cash budgets, balance sheets, and flexible budgeting. Tools that practices can use to analyze differences between budgets and actual experience also are presented.*

IMPORTANCE OF PLANNING

As the nature of the behavioral health practice changes, planning becomes critical. For some practices, prepaid services will become a larger percentage of revenues and present new challenges in accounting for the prepaid portion as well as the fee-for-service component. Additionally, the rapidly changing health care environment (i.e., technological and regulatory changes, the emergence of integrated delivery systems) has created many uncertainties for practitioners. Perhaps the most pronounced financial opportunity exists in newly developing systems that offer equity (ownership) stakes for its practitioners.

Although it is difficult to anticipate specific changes in the environment, from a broad-based perspective, general directions that behavioral health care policy will take in the near term can be forecasted to permit practices to plan pragmatically. Consultants to the behavioral health care field expect strong growth in managed behavioral health as market consolidation continues among providers (hospitals and practitioners), insurers, and public programs. The emergence and development of large integrated delivery systems offering a full continuum of care at capitated rates represent a significant market development. Each practice may choose how and whether to respond to such dynamics in its strategic plan.

SETTING GOALS AND STRATEGIC PLANNING

The planning process allows a practice to look forward and develop specific courses of action to achieve specified goals. All business activities are considered during planning. For example, determining what services to offer and determining staffing support levels are important to business planning.

Strategic planning is the creation of a long-term course of action to achieve goals; it usually spans periods of 5 years or more. Given the rapidly changing nature of health care, it is advisable that the strategic plan be reviewed and revised annually. Strategic plans set priorities for actions that include:

- future scope and span of services
- professional staffing levels
- financial policies
- marketing methods

Operational planning includes the development of short-term plans or tactics to achieve goals established in the long-term strategic plan. An operational plan supports the strategic plan and can cover time periods of a week, a month, a year, or more. Some operational planning objectives include determining staffing levels for the next month and setting the current month's target number of patient encounters.

Strategic and operational planning should occur, to some degree, in both solo practices and group practices. Obviously, the level of detail of the plan is commensurate with the size and complexity of the organization. Some solo practitioners do not see a need for a formal plan; however, the time invested in developing one will prove useful in the event a practice requires investment capital, wants to take in new partners, or considers merging with another practice. If further growth or mergers are not in a practice's future, a plan will still serve as a thought and provide guidance for maintaining the practice's viability.

COMPONENTS OF A STRATEGIC PLAN

There are three components to a strategic plan: the purpose statement, environmental analysis, and goals and objectives.

Purpose Statement

The first component of a strategic plan is a purpose statement; it defines the overall mission of the practice. The purpose may be defined either specifically or in general terms. For example, one practice might state that its purpose is "to provide our patients with the most appropriate care in the timeliest fashion." Another practice might state that its principal goal is "to increase the value of the practice's business for its stakeholders." A practice's statement defines why the practice is unique in the market.

The scope defines the practice's lines of business and geographical area of operation. An example statement of scope would be, "We are a group of behavioral health professionals providing adolescent services in the metro area."

Environmental Analysis

The second element of a strategic plan is an environmental analysis. A practice completes an environmental analysis as part of its strategic plan to systematically examine the conditions surrounding the practice and identify environmental factors affecting it. The objective is to discover the most influential factors, especially those beyond the practice's direct control. A thorough analysis might include an understanding of recent economic trends, changes in technology (i.e., outcomes measurement), demographic trends, sociopolitical trends (e.g., proposed privatization of Medicare/Medicaid), and legal/regulatory influences. This should reflect a general understanding of the market, and research in professional periodicals at a local library should be more than sufficient. Armed with this knowledge, the practice may elect to respond with specific actions.

Practitioners may also identify various concerns that can be addressed within the practice. There have been many recent changes in health care that may be included in the assessment, such as the growth of health maintenance organizations (HMOs), preferred provider organizations (PPOs), and other managed care arrangements, and changes in Medicare and Med-icaid. An environmental analysis includes consideration of patients, third-party payers, and other stakeholders.

Patients

A potential patient's knowledge level about the services provided by a behavioral health practice may range from extensive to nothing. There are a variety of reasons people seek behavioral health services. The information that patients receive about behavioral health services comes from a variety of sources: family, friends, teachers, school counselors, and clergy, to name a few. Patients may fail to differentiate the various types of pro-viders. For example, the terms "psychologist" and "psychiatrist" are often used interchangeably.

On the other hand, patients are becoming more involved in the health care decision-making process. "Report cards" are becoming more com-monplace, as are provider profiles. This information is becoming increas-ingly more available to patients and other third-party payers. In fact, these two initiatives were *driven* by payers' need to assess value in some measur-able terms. Practices may want to consider the implications of such initia-tives during the planning process. For example:

- Would expanding our efforts to educate the patient be worthwhile?
- Will an educated public require more or different behavioral health care services?
- How will the practice respond to changes in demand for the ser-vices noted above?

Insurers

Insurance companies have had a major impact on health care delivery in the past. In traditional fee-for-service health care, the insurance com-pany accepted the risk, changed an annual premium, and reimbursed pro-viders as services were rendered. As health care costs spiraled upward, there was great pressure to control costs. The current trend is to shift risk from insurers to providers, since providers ultimately make many of the decisions to spend health care dollars. In effect, provider groups that ac-cept full financial risk for providing capitated services are becoming "mi-cro" insurance companies.

The federal and state governments, through their Medicare and Med-icaid programs, also are influential third-party payers. The federal government has been trying to stem the rise in Medicare costs for several years. The creation and proliferation of diagnostic related groups (DRGs) for acute hospitalization and resource based relative value scales (RBRVSs) for clinical services have affected many aspects of health care delivery. These programs also influence the incentives for health care providers. Where emphasis used to be on acute and invasive treatments, it is now shifting toward wellness and prevention.

Local insurance trends may be considered in strategic planning. This information could come from a variety of sources, including on-line information (Internet), consultants, and locally published health care periodicals. Also, a practice might form its own focus group to solicit interview-type information from local providers. This, however, may be more time consuming. The state insurance commissioner's office also is an excellent source of free information.

- How much managed care exists in the local area?
- Are providers being unwillingly squeezed out of the fee-for-service market?
- Is there pressure to join a large network?

Goals and Objectives

After conducting an environmental assessment, a practice develops goals and objectives. Goals are broad long-term statements indicating what the practice wants to achieve. Objectives are short-term statements that operationalize the practice's goals, are more specific than goals, are measurable, and have definitive time horizons. Goals often spring from a set of shared values that exist among the members of the behavioral health practice. Goals should be reviewed from time to time but seldom changed. The goal-setting process is an integral part of the success of a practice.

How to Set Goals and Objectives

In order for a practice to set goals and objectives, its providers should address certain basic questions:

- What services will the practice offer?
- What patient groups will it serve?
- Does the practice wish to be a market leader, a market follower, or serve a unique and specialized market?

- How large (in terms of providers and office staff) does the practice want to be in the next 5 years?
- What changes in the national health care market will affect the practice?
- What changes in the local health care market will affect the practice?
- What is the expected impact of demographic trends on the practice (i.e., aging of the population, growth of single-parent families)?
- What is the impact of government regulation and/or legislation on the practice?

Based on the answers to these and other questions, the practice can develop several goal statements that become targets to attain. Next, the practice develops short- and medium-range objectives. The objectives cover 1- to 3-year time frames and are somewhat specific. They may represent quantitative variables (e.g., the number of patient sessions per professional) or qualitative variables (e.g., being on the leading edge of research in the industry). Objectives may be challenging yet realistically attainable. Some examples of variables that can be included in objectives are:

- patient encounters
- gross charges
- compensation
- capital acquisitions
- collection rates
- short-term resource balances
- market share
- return on investment

Gathering Input for Goal Setting in a Group Practice

One approach to goal setting in a solo, group, or facility practice is devising a questionnaire for the providers in the practice. It should be designed to ask pointed questions in an easy-to-answer format that focus on the basic issues of the practice. The questionnaire may ask providers to rank order or in some way prioritize their concerns about the practice. Table 1 lists sample questions that can be used to solicit provider input for various areas of the practice.

After each provider has responded, the practice decides on its goals—

TABLE 1   Sample Questions for Provider Input

Area	Questions
Facilities	What facilities are needed to meet current and future needs?
Professional services	What services will be offered?
Support staff	What are the personnel needs? What are their training needs? How can exceptional staff members be retained?
Finances	What financial resources are needed to accomplish the plans? What are the financial information reporting needs?
Marketing	What are the target market segments? What promotional and public relations activities will be pursued?
Productivity	What productivity levels are expected?
Management Information Systems	What are the information systems needs?
Social responsibility	What is the role of the practice in the health care community?

primary and secondary ones. Primary goals provide overall direction for the practice and are of a higher priority than secondary goals, which may be helpful but not critical to the success of the practice. Sample practice goals might include any one of the following:

- Achieve a 10% local market share in the geriatric behavioral health market.
- Have 30% of the practice be independent of third-party reimbursement.
- Grow to a practice of 10 psychologists within 5 years.

OPERATIONAL BUDGETS

The framework created by the practice's goals and objectives helps in creating operating plans for the near term. Again, operating plans are short-term plans to achieve goals. Objectives link sort-term operations plans with long-term goals. Operating budgets express these short-term plans in financial terms.

Budgeting requires a practice to plan in a systematic and focused way. Since budgets are short-term targets, tracked in dollars, practices usually allot specific time each year for the budget planning process. The process reflects the established goals and objectives of the organization. Small group and solo practices especially may benefit from formalization of the financial planning and budgeting processes.

The following section discusses budgeting from a broad perspective and tools for creating a comprehensive budget and a flexible budget.

Roles and Advantages of a Budget

A budget fulfills the following roles and provides advantages and benefits:

- Assists in the coordination and communication of short-term plans, which increase in importance as the practice grows.
- Authorizes staff members to acquire and use resources during the coming period to cultivate new activities.
- Provides the practice with a progress gauge and tracking system.
- Allows a practice to anticipate conditions so that positive situations can be capitalized on and negative ones minimized.
- Creates benchmarks to control ongoing actions and develop criteria for evaluating practice performance at all levels.

Parts of a Comprehensive Budget

A comprehensive budget is based on a projection of revenues and expenses as well as a number of financial statements that a practice may already produce on a regular basis. Each step is explained in later sections of this chapter. A comprehensive budget consists of two main sections: (1) planning and control mechanisms for cash and (2) a formal budget made up of a profit plan, cash budget, capital expenditures budget, and projected balance sheet.

Preparation of a Comprehensive Budget

This discussion of a comprehensive budget uses the commonly accepted accrual accounting method. The cash basis method is not covered in detail here. A practice's accountant can give advice on which method would be most appropriate.

The accrual accounting method requires a practice to note when it has incurred an obligation for debts. It also requires that revenues be noted at the time services are provided; that is, the provider notes income for patient visits when the services are rendered, not when the patient or insurer actually pays the provider at some later date. Three portions of a comprehensive budget are the profit plan, the cash budget, and the balance sheet.

Budgeting Revenues

Projecting revenues is key to the development of an operating budget because without knowing how much revenue a practice can expect to earn, the practice's ability to meet its financial goals (e.g., income, purchase a building, expand the number of providers) cannot be determined. All expenses, cash distribution, cash flow, and capital expenditure projections depend on an accurate projection of operating revenues.

There are various methods for estimating future revenues. They include the following.

- *Demand estimates.* These estimates involve a determination of potential demand for the services offered by the group or practice. Demand calculations are useful for marketing strategies and long-range planning functions. Because several methods of estimation are available, an estimate is subject to potential error. However, an estimate can be useful for long-term planning and when providing prepaid services to HMO patients.

Periodic assessment of future demand for services supports planning for a practice's size and rate of growth. The method is similar to determining a share of the market. Estimating demand requires three types of data:

- Demographic characteristics of the geographical area (check local/federal government offices, local library, or on-line computer services). For example, if a practice provides child behavioral health services, census data will indicate the growth of this population by age group and county.
- Patient usage rates for each specialty or service (make assumptions based on practice experience). For example, utilization data for child mental health services are typically measured in inpatient days per 1,000 or outpatient visits per 1,000. This information is not, however, always conveniently available. Two possible sources include any managed behavioral health plan that the practice currently does business with or a quali-

fied consultant that has this information specific for the population and area served by the practice.

- Potential market share that the practice expects or desires (based on practice goals and strategic plans).

For example, a practice specializing in geriatrics assumes the average patient will have five visits annually at $100 per visit. If the practice wants to achieve 5% of the local geriatric market, it estimates it will see 600 of the 12,000 geriatric patients currently being treated in the local area, for an annual revenue of $300,000 (600 x 5 x $100). Again, this information is generally limited to the aforementioned sources, but it is available.

- *Past activity levels* (see Exhibit 1). This is another method of estimating demand that assumes recent past numbers of patient encounters are the best measure of future demand. Known changes in the practice (e.g., addition/retirement of psychologists, fee schedule changes) are projected. This method is generally used by fee-for-service practices and assumes that psychologist time is the limiting resource on patient demand. Be careful when annualizing encounter data to account for low-activity months in the overall budget.

Exhibit 1   Revenue Projection Based on Past Activity

Month	No. of Encounters Previous Year	Projected No. of Encounters	Fee per Encounter ($)	Projected Revenue ($)
1	200	210	100	2,100
2	190	200	100	2,000
3	220	230	100	2,300
4	200	210	100	2,100
5	190	200	100	2,000
6	180	190	100	1,900
7	170	180	100	1,800
8	210	220	100	2,200
9	220	230	100	2,300
10	230	240	100	2,400
11	240	250	100	2,500
12	240	250	100	2,500
Total	2,500	2,620	100	262,000

• *Estimate of the number of patient encounters/visits.* In a group practice this estimate is based on what is planned by each psychologist during the budget period. The fee schedule is applied to the expected number of visits, and budgeted production can be determined for each provider, as shown in Exhibit 2.

Exhibit 2   Projected Patient Visits Revenue Worksheet

	No. of Fee-for-Service Visits	Total Fee-for-Service Charges[a]	No. of Prepaid Visits	Total ($) Prepaid Charges[b]	Total No. of Visits	Total Charges ($)
1	200	20,000	30	2,550	230	25,550
2	220	22,000	20	1,700	240	23,700
3	210	21,000	10	850	220	21,850
4	190	19,000	20	1,700	210	20,700
5	200	20,000	30	2,550	230	22,550
6	150	15,000	20	1,700	170	16,700
7	230	23,000	20	1,700	250	24,700
8	210	21,000	20	850	220	21,850
9	220	22,000	20	1,700	240	23,700
10	200	20,000	20	1,700	220	21,700
11	190	19,000	20	1,700	210	20,700
Total						243,700

[a]Fee-for-service average is $100.
[b]Discounted fee-for-service is $85 (85% of $100)

Budgeting Expenses

Estimating expenses is the next step in developing a budget. It entails estimating costs, which are either fixed or variable. Fixed costs (such as salaries and overhead) do not change as the number of patient visits changes. Variable costs (such as supplies) change according to the number of patient visits.

• The following formula describes the relationship between costs and patient visits:
  Total costs = fixed costs + (variable cost per visit × number of visits)
• By expressing costs as fixed or variable, they can be calculated for

any level of patient visits. Budgeting allows a practice to project costs when developing an operating budget and profit plan. At the end of the period, actual costs can be compared with the amounts budgeted by using the actual number of patient visits experienced for the period.

Exhibit 3 classifies typical expenses by behavior pattern and shows the flexible budgeting formula based on last year's costs. To project fixed costs, they are identified as committed or programmed in the exhibit. *Committed fixed costs* are based on long-range decisions and are typically unchanged for long periods of time. These costs include depreciation, lease expenses, insurance, and property taxes. *Programmed fixed costs* arise from short-term plans. These costs include staff salaries, benefits, repairs, and marketing costs. Flexible budgeting is covered in greater detail later in this chapter.

Preparation of a Profit Plan

A profit plan integrates budgeted revenues and expenses to show the net income for individual psychologists or the total practice in the case of

---

Exhibit 3   Cost Classification Worksheet

Costs	Cost Type	Flexible Budget, Year 1 (average month)	Expected Changes, Year 2
Psychologists' salaries	Programmed fixed	$10,000	Increase on 1/1 to $12,000
Psychologists' benefits	Programmed fixed	(a) 30% of salaries (b) 3% of salaries for professional development	(a) No change (b) Increase to 5% of salaries
Staff salaries	Programmed fixed	$2,500	10% increase
Staff benefits	Programmed fixed	30% of salaries	No change
Supplies	Variable	$1 per visit	No change
Equipment rentals	Committed fixed	$200 per month	No change

a group practice. For purposes of planning, controlling, and reporting, the profit plan and performance reports can be related to individual providers in the group.

Individual Provider Profit Plan

Using data from Exhibit 1 and cost behavior pattern information, a profit plan is developed, as shown in Exhibit 4. Only expenses directly traceable to the individual provider are included in the plan. Revenues are estimated for each month of the first quarter and totaled. Expenses are similarly listed. The contribution to income is the difference between total projected revenues and expenses.

Many groups entering prepaid arrangements establish accountability for their prepaid contracts. Each service area is given a credit for patient encounters to provide individual psychologists with a revenue measure. In a prepaid practice, revenues are the capitated payments from the HMO. Expenses include the cost of service provided to prepaid patients (fee-for-service equivalents) and the cost of outside referrals. (Refer to the APA Practitioner's Toolbox Series volume *Contracting on a Capitated Basis: Managing Risk for Your Practice* for further details.)

Aggregate Profit Plans

A profit plan forecasts whether total patient revenues will cover expenses and provide practitioners with a satisfactory income. Patient encounters and net revenues are totaled for the whole practice. Expenses are presented separately by provider. Alternatively, common costs can be deducted from the contributions of each provider.

If the providers are dissatisfied with the results, the profit plan can be prepared using different levels of patient visits and expenses. Individual providers, expenses, or fee schedules may require adjustment to reach a satisfactory outcome.

PREPARING A CASH BUDGET

The next part of a comprehensive budget is a cash budget, which shows the expected sources and uses of cash for the coming period (usually 1 year). The cash budget is prepared after the profit plan is completed. A profit plan and cash budget can be kept current by adding new monthly

Exhibit 4   Sample Profit Plan

	January	February	Quarter 1 March	Year Total	Total
Fee-for-service net revenue	$20,000	$20,000	$21,000	$63,000	$222,000
Prepaid gross charges (fee-for-service equivalent)	2,550	1,700	850	5,100	21,700
Total revenue	**$22,550**	**$21,700**	**$21,850**	**$68,100**	**$240,700**
Operating Expenses					
Psychologists' salaries	$10,000	$10,000	$10,000	$30,000	$120,000
Psychologists' benefits	2,300	2,300	2,300	6,900	27,600
Staff salaries	2,500	2,500	2,500	7,500	30,000
Staff benefits	500	500	500	1,500	6,000
Supplies	927	1,025	1,008	2,930	12,379
Equipment rental	200	200	200	600	2,400
Liability insurance	400	400	400	1,200	4,800
Total expenses	**$16,827**	**$16,925**	**$16,908**	**$50,660**	**$203,179**
Contribution to income	$5,723	$6,775	$4,942	$17,440	$37,521

figures at the end of each month and new quarterly figures at the end of each quarter. To complete a cash budget, a practice collects the following data:

- beginning cash balance
- projected cash received from patients or other sources
- projected cash to be used for operating expenses
- projected cash expenditures for capital acquisitions
- projected cash to be borrowed and repaid
- ending cash balance

An example of a cash budget is shown in Exhibit 5.

PREPARING A BALANCE SHEET

The final step in completing a comprehensive budget is the creation of a projected balance sheet, sometimes called a Statement of Assets and Liabilities. A sample balance sheet is given in chapter 4.

The main function of a balance sheet is to link the planning docu-

---

Exhibit 5   Cash Budget

	January	February	March
Cash collected from patients	$17,000	$16,000	$18,000
- Cash used for operating expenses	15,500	10,000	10,000
= Cash increase from patient visits	$ 1,500	$ 6,000	$ 8,000
+ Beginning cash balance	10,000	10,800	21,000
= Ending cash balance before other cash transactions	11,500	16,800	29,000
+ Cash from nonoperating sources (e.g., investments)	100	0	5,000
- Payments on debt	800	800	800
+ Purchase of short-term investments	0	0	0
= Ending cash balance before borrowing	10,800	16,000	33,200
+ Borrowing to maintain minimum balance	0	5,000	0
= Ending cash balance	$10,800	$21,000	$33,200

ments and detail the practice's financial position at the end of the budget period. The balance sheet is a snapshot view of the practice's financial position. A practice that maintains active cash management, supply control, and collections functions may find that its projected and actual balance sheets closely match.

USING THE BUDGET

A budget is a target based on an informed estimate of likely future events. When budgets are compared to actual revenues and expenses, deviations may occur. Although a practice attempts to reach its planned number of patient encounters, actual expenses and revenues are rarely identical to the planned amounts. Causes of variance may include:

- more or fewer patient encounters
- changes in pricing for fees and/or in expenses
- more or less effective use of budgeted resources
- loss of a managed care contract or other change in cash flow collections

A large concern in using a budget is accounting for the variances that arise. If changes in patient visits are accompanied by changes in resource utilization (e.g., a provider took a 3-month sabbatical), it may incorrectly be assumed that the change in patient encounters is causing inefficiencies. This is where the concept of flexible budgeting becomes a factor.

THE FLEXIBLE BUDGET

The comprehensive budget already described can be prepared in two ways: a static form, where patient encounters are assumed to be unchanging, or a flexible form, where different volume levels are accounted for. Other than volume, both budgets have identical assumptions. The flexible budget is prepared as a series of static budgets, each reflecting a different level of patient visits.

Estimating patient encounters is difficult for any health care organization. The volume of activity depends on a number of internal and external forces, some of which are outside a practice's control. Fluctuations in planned activity levels will cause variances from budgeted revenues and expenses. Flexible budgeting provides an excellent approach to planning and performance reporting when it is difficult to estimate future volume and when costs vary in response to volume changes.

Flexible budgeting, when used for performance reporting purposes, allows practices to evaluate how budgeted costs compare with actual patient encounters. It is important because it helps a practice determine if it is meeting its goals and if the goals are realistic. Table 2 outlines the advantages and disadvantages of static and flexible budgets.

Requirements for Flexible Budgeting

In a group practice each provider consumes some of the practice's resources, typically time, while providing services to patients. The practice may use the unit-of-service approach to costing. The simplest measure of resource utilization and related costs is a patient encounter. Each patient encounter equals one unit of service. Computing the average cost of resources used per visit equals total practice costs divided by total practice encounters. The result is a single number that is an overall measure of the average cost of resources used to produce one patient encounter; however, there is no distinction regarding the intensity, effort, or expertise of each encounter. For example, 1 hour of therapy equals 1 hour of psychological testing.

TABLE 2   Advantages and Disadvantages of Static and Flexible Budgets

	Static Budget	Flexible Budget
Advantages	• Simple, easy to understand • Can be prepared manually • Requires less time to complete than flexible budget • Meaningful tool if actual activity is near budgeted level	• Can be adjusted to reflect actual activity levels • Easier to accurately analyze variances from budgeted to actual
Disadvantages	• Cannot be easily adjusted to reflect actual activity level • If actual activity level varies greatly from budget, it is difficult to analyze discrepancies • Variances are blamed on volume changes rather than other controllable factors	• Requires more time and resources to complete • Usually requires use of computer • Requires higher level of sophistication by administrative personnel and providers to properly use the budget

An example of unit-of-service costing for a psychological practice is as follows:

- Determine the total number of patient encounters
  Total encounters = 1,500
- Determine the total direct costs
  Total costs = $127,500
- Divide total direct costs by total encounter
  $127,500 ÷ 1,500 = $85 per patient encounter

Flexible Budget Variances

Once a flexible budget has been established, it becomes invaluable in analyzing the practice's performance. At the end of each month or reporting period, actual expenses can be compared to the budget prediction of expenses.

To accomplish this, the budgeted volumes are replaced with the actual volumes. The budgeted variable unit-of-service costs are multiplied by the actual patient volume to obtain the true variable costs. This amount is added to the budgeted fixed costs to arrive at the "flexed" budgeted costs, which can be compared with actual costs.

- Actual variable costs + actual fixed costs = "flexed" budgeted costs (i.e., budget costs accounting for volume)

Any difference between flexed budget costs and actual costs relates to how well resources were matched to the level of output. As the year progresses, the flexible budget can be modified to incorporate actual changes in costs (e.g., increased staff wages, increased utility rates).

TOOLS OF ANALYZING VARIANCES

A practice can use ratios and other financial analyses to determine if it is meeting its financial goals. Some important questions a practice may want to answer include:

- What are the financial consequences if the psychologists' salaries are increased?
- How many sessions are necessary to cover the bills each month?
- How much money does the practice make from each service?

Consequence of Increasing Salaries

To determine the consequences of increasing psychologists' salaries, the practice can determine its contribution margin, which demonstrates the effect of an increase or decrease in patient volume on a practice's income. Contribution margin equals patient revenues minus variable costs and fixed expenses. Deducting fixed costs and expenses from the contribution margin gives the operating income or loss. For example:

Annual gross revenue	$243,000
Variable costs	40,000
Contribution margin	203,000
Fixed costs	183,000
Operating income	$ 20,000

The contribution margin can also be expressed as a percentage:

$$\text{Contribution margin ratio} = \frac{\text{Gross revenue} - \text{variable costs}}{\text{Sales}}$$

Example

$$83\% = \frac{\$243,000 - \$40,000}{\$243,000}$$

This ratio indicates the percentage of each dollar of revenue that is available to cover fixed costs and provide operating income. If psychologists' salaries are raised, the fixed expenses will be higher and the practice's operating income will be lower. To maintain the same level of operating income, the practice must see more patients or reduce its variable costs. Calculating the contribution margin can also help the practice answer questions related to other expenses, such as the effect of moving to a more costly office location.

How Much Money Does the Practice Make From Each Service?

Psychologists may wish to know the financial value of each additional service. For example, a psychologist might be paid $100 for a patient visit, but how much of that contributes to the practice's net income? To determine this answer, providers can compute the unit contribution margin, which is the money available from each patient visit to cover fixed costs and provide profits to the practice. For example, if the average fee per patient is $100 and the average variable cost per patient is $35, the unit contribution margin is $65.

How Many Sessions and What Kinds of Services Are Needed to Cover the Bills?

Some providers, particularly those starting practices, are most concerned with being able to pay their bills each month. To accomplish this, providers can compute their practice's break-even point, which is the level of operations at which revenues and costs are equal. At this point, the practice will neither make a profit nor experience a loss, but all expenses will be covered. For example, if a behavioral health practice were trying to decide whether to begin offering marriage and family therapy in addition to individual therapy, it can use a breakeven analysis to determine if it should hire another psychologist.

Break-even analysis using equations

The break-even point is computed by dividing fixed costs by the unit contribution margin:

$$\text{Break-even point for patient encounters} = \frac{\text{Fixed costs}}{\text{Contribution margin per encounter}}$$

For example,
average fee per patient = $100
variable cost = $35
unit contribution = $65
fixed costs = $65,000
break-even point is $65,000 ÷ $65 = 1,000 patient visits

Break-even analysis using graphs

The break-even point as shown in Figure 1, is the point at which the revenue line crosses the total costs line. Figure 2 shows another form of break-even, known as the profit volume chart. Rather than using revenue, the break-even point is shown to be the intersection of the contribution margin line and the fixed cost line. The points along the contribution margin line are the amount of income at any given number of patient visits (patient visits x unit contribution).

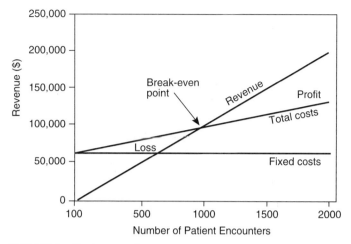

FIGURE 1   Break-even chart.

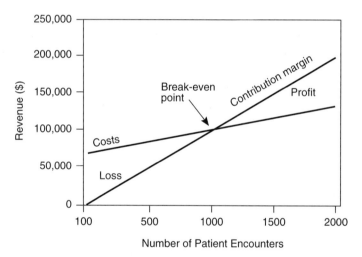

FIGURE 2   Profit-volume chart.

These figures are useful in showing a practice's possible courses of action. If a practice is not reaching the break-even point or is dissatisfied with its profit level, it can change any of three things.

1. Increase the fee per patient encounter, as shown in Figure 3. In this case the number of patient encounters needed for a practice to break even is lower, and each addition encounter increases the profits.

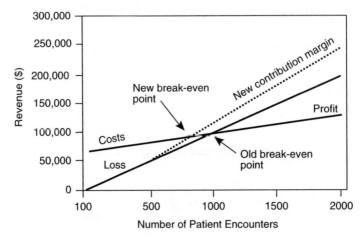

FIGURE 3   Profit-volume chart.

2. Increase the number of patient encounters (see Figure 4). In this case the cost and contribution margin lines do not change, but, as the practice increases its number of patient encounters, the level of profits increases.
3. Decrease costs, as shown in Figure 5. Here, the entire contribution margin line moves, which results in an earlier break-even point (i.e., fewer patient sessions are required to cover the bills).

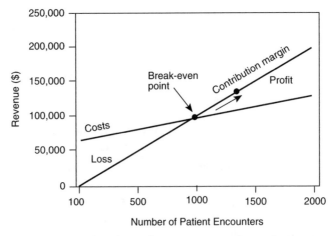

FIGURE 4   Profit-volume chart: increasing volume of encounters.

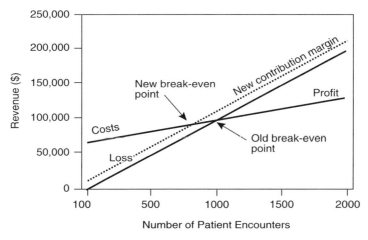

FIGURE 5   Profit-volume chart: decreasing fixed costs.

Financial Analysis for a Capitated Practice

In a capitated practice the patients are enrolled in an HMO and pay a monthly premium. The practice receives a monthly payment per person and, in turn, provides necessary services. If the number of enrolled patients is used as the measure of activity, the break-even chart will look as shown in Figure 6.

For a prepaid practice to increase profits, it must do one of three things:

- Increase the per-patient capitation rate
- Reduce operating costs
- Increase the number of enrolled patients

The capitation practice is rewarded for efficient use of resources. Anything it can do to reduce the use of resources while maintaining quality will increase the practice's income. (Refer to the APA Practitioner's Toolbox Series volume *Contracting on a Capitated Basis: Managing Risk for Your Practice* for more information on prepaid contracts.)

SUMMARY

Planning and budgeting are important aspects of running a successful psychological practice. Planning is the process a practice uses to develop a course of action to attain its goals. A budget is a financial framework that

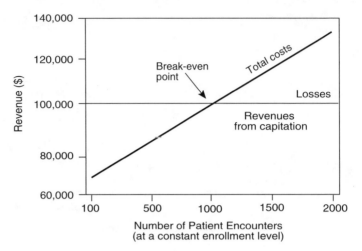

FIGURE 6   Break-even chart: prepaid practice.

a practice creates to help achieve its objectives. Going through the process of creating a strategic plan requires practitioners to think beyond daily activities, to separate themselves from the distractions of the moment, and to think about their practice in a larger context. The budgeting process provides a practice with valuable financial information. It helps the practice discern how it will specifically meet some of its goals and objectives. In addition, it gives providers a tool for determining if its goals are realistic.

2

Types of Financing

T HIS CHAPTER EXPLORES *the various types of financing available to practices. After completing the planning and budgeting process, the next step for a practice is to select the type of financing that best meets its objectives. There are several different types of financing, each differing in cost, flexibility, and restraints. Commercial banks, finance companies, insurance carriers, and leasing companies are examples of institutions that provide financing. In addition, practices may use internal sources and equity capital, which is supplied by providers, venture capitalists, and others.*

Capital is an enabling factor that allows a practice to begin or to grow. Capital requirements determined in the budgeting process drive the staffing and technical resource decisions that allow a practice to expand its ability to provide services. Providers may need to have a rudimentary understanding of financial matters appropriate to the size of the practice. Larger practices may employ an office manager who handles the billing and accounting; a designated provider is often responsible for determining whether the office manager is performing properly. In smaller groups and individual practices, an understanding of finances may be more important because the practice's survival may depend on a provider's ability to budget and acquire necessary financing.

It may help providers to know that, while the health care industry is undergoing significant changes, so is the banking industry. In the past, many loans were secured on a provider's word and a handshake. Today, banks still welcome the business that health care providers bring, but they are no longer permitted to rely on a provider's word. Many lending institutions approach financing in a more cautious manner and require all borrowers to present detailed and sophisticated business plans before approving a line of credit or a loan.

WHY A PRACTICE MAY NEED CAPITAL

There are four main reasons a practice may need capital: to start a practice, to buy/lease equipment, to buy real estate, and to acquire another practice. Like any other business, a behavioral health practice needs capital to operate. Capital requirements vary depending on the stage of business a practice is in as well as the size of the practice. For example, launching a practice may require more funds than expanding one. Capital needs are also driven by the scope of services offered and the level of risk aversion of the borrower. Risk aversion is the level of risk a provider is willing to assume. The more risk averse a provider is, the more conservative the financing approach may be. Each financial need might be best supported by a different method of financing.

Financing Decisions Using Debt or Equity

There are many financing instruments that a growing practice might use: lines of credit, term loans, mortgage notes, common stock. All of these options can be categorized either as debt or equity.
- *Debt financing* is defined as a practice incurring an obligation to repay the funds it receives. There is no change in the ownership structure of the practice when a debt is incurred. Examples of debt financing are a term loan, lease, or mortgage note.
- *Equity financing* is defined by a practice giving a portion of its ownership to whomever is providing the capital. Examples of equity financing would be a general partnership or stock offering.

Table 3 summarizes the financing instruments available, the typical uses of each instrument, and what size practice each instrument best suits.

Every practice is faced with establishing a capital structure for its financing base. In other words, what portion of the total value of the practice will be debt and what portion equity? Each has advantages and disadvantages. It may sometimes be necessary to use debt to finance an entire practice. Although debt is less expensive than equity, as a practice's debt rises, the risk associated with the debt increases, because banks and other lending institutions become concerned about the drain of cash devoted to paying interest on the debt. In addition, as the amount of debt increases,

TABLE 3   Types of Financing Instruments

Financing Instrument	Practice Start-up	Minor Equipment	Real Estate	Practice Acquisition
Debt financing				
Short-term (<1 year)		Solo, small, large		
Medium-term (1–8 years	Solo	Solo, small, large		Solo, small, large
Long-term (3–30 years)			Solo, small, large	
Lease (2–8 years)	Solo	Solo, small, large	Solo, small	Solo
Internal sources				
Operations		Small, large		Large
Retained earnings			Small, large	Large
Equity				
General partnership	Small, large		Small, large	Large
Limited partnership			Solo, small, large	
Stock corporation	Solo, small, large		Small, large	
Joint venture			Solo, small, large	

Note. Solo = solo practitioner; small = small group practice (2–10 providers); large = large group practice (more than 10 providers).

the likelihood the practice will fail also increases. Depending on the organization of the practice and the type of debt, the provider may be personally liable for the practice's debts.

Financing a practice without using any debt may not be the best solution either. If providers do not supply all the equity, they may have to relinquish a share of their business to outside interests. If they do supply all the equity, they retain full ownership. It may be a problem, however, for some psychologists to commit to providing that amount of money. New providers may have personal debt incurred during their education.

The age of a practice also affects the choice of debt or equity financing. In the first few years of a practice, equity financing may be the best choice. As the practice grows, establishes itself in the community, and appears to be less risky, debt financing may become more readily available.

Each provider or practice decides on a capital structure. Most practices adopt a combined debt/equity structure, with the mix varying with the degree of risk the practice is willing to assume. Providers who are risk averse may not want a large loan to repay, while others may be perfectly comfortable financing their practices with a large amount of debt.

DEBT FINANCING

Debt financing is available with many options. Table 4 summarizes some of the relevant attributes of debt.

TABLE 4   Debt Financing Attributes

	Interest Rate	Term (length)	Security Required?
Sort-term loan	Variable	<1 year	No
Medium-term loan	Fixed or variable	1–8 years	Yes/equipment
Long-term loan	Fixed or variable	8–30 years	Yes/real estate
Lease	Fixed	2–8 years	Yes/equipment

A fixed interest rate does not change over the life of the loan. A variable rate can move higher or lower, but usually goes higher because lenders often set the initial rate low in order to entice borrowers.

Security refers to the collateral that lenders sometimes require to make a loan. If no security is required (an unsecured loan), the provider simply signs papers promising to repay the loan. If security is required, the provider is required to pledge something of value (e.g., building, land, or other asset) and a guarantee of repayment. If the provider defaults on a secured loan, the lender may seize or repossess the pledged asset.

The lender's financial manager can influence the term of the loan, payment arrangements, type of interest rate, interest level, and collateral. Many lenders are accustomed to working with health care providers and understand the special circumstances that may affect a provider's ability to pay. For example, a psychologist setting up a solo practice may need 6 months or longer to generate a steady cash flow. Initial loan payments may be delayed or reduced for that time until the psychologist is earning a steady income and cash flow is established. Another way to accommodate a fledgling practice is to structure the payments such that the provider pays only the interest for a period of time. Later, when the practice is established, both interest and principal repayments will be made or a balloon payment will be used. A balloon payment is a large portion or the entire principal due at the end of the loan.

Debt financing is typically characterized by the term. Short-term loans require payment within 1 year, medium-term loans have a 2- to 8-year time horizon, and long-term loans encompass an 8- to 30-year time frame.

Short-Term Financing

Short-term financing refers to loans that have a repayment period of less than 1 year. There are several variables that define the loan:

- Demand note (subject to payment when the lender requests)
- Promissory note (specified date for repayment)
- Fixed principal (amount that is borrowed is fixed)
- Fluctuating principal (amount that is borrowed may change)

One type of short-term credit is a *line of credit*, which establishes a dollar amount that the lender is willing to extend. A line of credit may be predicated on certain conditions being met. The lender may be willing to provide the practice with an agreed-upon maximum amount, which the practice has the discretion to draw upon as needed. Interest is charged on the amount actually owed (not the credit line limit). The lender also might charge a fee to maintain a credit line.

Revolving credit is another short-term instrument that assures a line of credit with a maturity of up to 3 years with an option to convert any of the loan to a term loan at the end of the credit period.

Practices usually incur short-term financing to provide working capital. *Working capital* is defined as the amount of cash required to operate the practice for a specified time period, such as 6 months. Working capital is used to fund payroll, supplies, utilities, and rent until patients are billed and revenue is collected. Because of the fluid nature of these requirements, short-term loans may have a flexible repayment schedule that varies according to the practice's working capital needs. For example, as the balance of accounts receivable increases, the loan balance may rise as well.

When evaluating a practice's request for short-term loans, a lender is concerned with short-run cash flow rather than long-term changes in net worth or long-term profitability through successful management and operations. Therefore, the lender examines a practice's cash flow projections and other assurances that the practice can repay its debt through cash generated from patient encounters.

Interest rates on short-term loans may fluctuate according to general economic conditions. Most banks use the prime interest rate—the rate banks charge their most creditworthy clients—and other indices as a basis for floating interest charges. This allows interest rates to vary, thus minimizing the bank's risk. When the prime rate or other index increases, the interest rates on other loans increase automatically. The difference between the prime rate and the rate the bank charges a practice depends on several factors:

- Creditworthiness of the practice
- Size of the loan
- Collateral used to secure the loan
- Relationship of the practice and the bank

Banks and other lenders often require practices to maintain a minimum balance on account at their institutions. These are termed *compensating balances*, and the minimum requirement depends on the competitive conditions in the loan market and may be subject to negotiation. Compensating balance amounts may be up to 10 to 20% of a loan's balance. The effect of these balances on a practice is to raise the effective interest rate of the loan if the practice must maintain a higher balance than it ordinarily would, as shown below:

Loan amount: $50,000
Interest rate: 12%
Compensating balance requirement: 10%
Effective interest rate: 13.33%

In this example, the practice, rather than having the use of $50,000, now has only $45,000 available to it because it must keep $5,000 in the bank as the compensating balance requirement ($50,000 × 10%). The effective interest rate is now 13.3% ($6,000 in annual interest/$45,000 in available cash), rather than the 12% stated in the loan document.

MEDIUM-TERM LOANS

Medium-term loan financing refers to debt with a repayment term of 1 to 8 years. Generally, these loans are secured by specific tangible assets such as equipment or leasehold improvements. The length of the loan is determined by the asset being financed. Equipment financing is usually structured such that the term of the loan coincides with the life of the equipment. For example, if a practice finances the purchase of office equipment, including computers and furniture, that is expected to last 5 years, the term of the loan will likely be 5 years as well.

Loan repayments normally consist of even installments paid over the life of the loan; however, a practice may negotiate specific accommodations to match expected cash flow. As with short-term debt, medium-term debt also may allow a practice to pay interest only for a specified period of time while deferring repayment of the principal.

To protect the bank against default, most medium-term loans include an acceleration clause that stipulates immediate repayment of the entire principal upon default of any payment. Interest rates on medium-term loans vary depending on the credit risk associated with the practice. Fixed-rate loans usually have higher interest rates than loans with variable rates initially, but over time variable rates may become higher than fixed rates depending on the index selected. Variable-rate loans may be tied to the prime lending rate with upper and lower limits (termed *collar*) or an upper interest rate limit only (termed *cap*). For example, a variable-rate loan may begin at 8% with a lower limit of 6% and an upper limit of 10%.

There are several factors that determine the interest rate of a medium-term loan:

- Loan amount
- Practice's credit rating
- Maturity date (term of loan)
- Relationship between the bank and the practice

The medium-term interest rate is usually slightly higher than the short-term rate and may require a compensating balance of up to 10 or 20%. Usually, a bank would expect a practice to use the assets being financed as collateral for a loan. If the practice is purchasing new equipment, manufacturers will offer financing arrangements. The bank or other lender usually retains the option of repossessing the equipment in the event the practice defaults on the loan.

LONG-TERM LOANS

Long-term loans—debts with terms greater than 8 years—may be used to finance the purchase of real estate, buildings, and other asset. This debt instrument usually involves making installment payments. Mortgages, which are devices that allow a practice to borrow money by pledging real estate as security, have three characteristics:

- the lender's interest in the property ends when the loan is fully paid,
- the lender has a right to foreclose on the mortgage if the practice defaults, and
- the practice has a right to redeem or regain the property.

If for some reason the practice must sell the asset, the lender holding the mortgage has either first, second, or third claim on it. *Claim* refers to the order the lender stands in relation to other creditors.

Repayment of these loans requires periodic installments. As is the case with short- and medium-term loans, mortgages also may have interest-only payments followed by a balloon payment as the final repayment. Both fixed- and variable-rate mortgages are available with terms from 15 to 30 years for a mortgage and shorter terms for loans requiring a balloon payment.

A lender considers several factors when determining the contract terms of a long-term loan:

- the practice's net earning power (i.e., the amount of money it is likely to earn throughout its life, not just its short-term cash flow);
- the capability of the professionals in the practice; and
- the long-term prospects of both the practice and the health care industry.

LEASE FINANCING

Leasing is a financing alternative for acquiring the use of equipment without a large down payment. This type of financing is provided by banks, insurance companies, and specialized lease companies. The two most common variations of leases are operating and finance leases. An *operating lease*, which is a rental agreement with a shorter term than the expected life of the asset, is usually used for office space, cars, and office furniture. The assets do not become the property of the practice. A *finance lease* has terms that usually equal the expected life of the asset being financed. Finance leases are longer than operating leases and may provide for a bargain purchase option at the end of the lease period. Finance leases are very similar to conventional loans. One of the major decisions faced by behavioral health practices is deciding whether to lease or purchase equipment.

Advantages of Leasing

- Leasing eliminates the large down payment often required in a purchase. This frees funds to be used for other things by the practice. A down payment may amount to 20% of the purchase price, while a lease is 100% financed.
- A lease is often easier to obtain than other instruments because the leasing company continues to own the equipment.
- A lease limits the risk of the equipment becoming obsolete. Computer systems are examples of assets that become obsolete quickly.
- A practice is not usually responsible for servicing leased equipment, reducing both risks and maintenance costs.
- A lease need not be reported as a liability which may allow the practice to obtain more credit.

Disadvantages of Leasing

- Leasing is usually more costly than purchasing because the organization providing the lease retains the risk of ownership.
- A practice cannot depreciate the asset for tax purposes because it does not own the equipment.
- The manufacturer providing the lease may place restrictions on its use or charge extra for excessive use, such as a monthly mileage limit on a leased car.

EQUITY FINANCING

Equity financing involves transferring ownership interest in the practice. Funds obtained from issuing equity may be contributed by psychologists currently in the practice and/or new psychologists who join the group. If new psychologists contribute, the ownership interest of the existing psychologist-owners is diluted unless they contribute additional capital to retain their ownership percentage. There are several ways to obtain equity financing: through partnerships, corporations, and joint ventures. The discussion that follows is not meant to be a complete one on the topic of equity. Rather, it is meant to introduce the topic as a way of thinking about financing. A provider should consult with an accountant and/or attorney before making any final decisions.

Limited Partnerships

A limited partnership may be an appropriate vehicle for financing a behavioral health practice because such a partnership allows passive investors to join with a general partner in an investment without forcing the general partner to release control and without subjecting the passive investors to risks other than those associated with the investment. The limited partners provide funds without having any management responsibilities. The general partner manages the partnership. In a behavioral health practice the psychologists would be the general partners and an outside investor would be the limited partner. The psychologists run the practice and the outside investor, in return for money invested, receives income but has no voice in how the practice is managed.

Limited partnerships are well suited to behavioral health practices for financing equipment and real estate because they are formed with a limited scope and duration. Investors purchase units of interest in amounts set forth in an agreement and share in the profit of the partnership according to the agreement. Psychologists who are general partners are legally bound to manage the practice to the best of their ability (called *fiduciary responsibility*) but may have a much smaller financial investment than the limited partners. Sometimes the general partner contributes services as opposed to cash for its interest.

Corporations

A corporation is a legal entity that is separate and distinct from its owners and managers. A corporation has an unlimited life, which means it can continue after its original owners are gone. A corporation also permits easy transfer of ownership because ownership is divided into shares of stock that can be bought and sold. Finally, a corporation provides limited liability., If a corporation cannot repay its obligations, the owners are not held personally liable for repayment. Potential losses are limited to the amount of investment in the stock.

Setting up a corporation is more difficult than setting up a partnership or solo practice. A corporation requires a charter and bylaws. The charter states the name of the practice, the type of activity it will pursue, the amount of capital stock, the number of directors, and the names of the directors. The bylaws are a set of rules that state how directors will be elected, if current shareholders have first rights to purchase new shares, and other conditions.

The relative advantages and disadvantages of the aforementioned legal entities, including discussions of tax and governance issues, can be found in the APA Practitioner's Toolbox Series volume *Building a Group Practice: Creating a Shared Vision for Success*. It is strongly recommended that outside counsel is sought for guidance in these matters.

Table 5 compares the three types of equity a practice can have.

JOINT VENTURES

A joint venture is an organization formed by several entities to accomplish business goals that could not be achieved by an individual entity. A joint venture is formed for a defined period of time and for a limited purpose; it allows a practice to join forces with other organizations in accessing capital, equipment, technology, human resources, or markets.

In legal terms, a joint venture can be structured like a corporation, general partnership, or limited partnership. The organization chosen depends on the nature of the alliance, the risk involved, and tax considerations.

Prior to entering into a joint venture, an evaluation of the opportunity is made from the standpoint of the venture fitting into the overall business plan of the practice. Legal issues may also need to be resolved, such as:

- Determining who controls the venture
- Federal and state licensing and accreditation issues
- Antitrust implications
- Status of legislation regarding referrals and ownership issues

One recent phenomenon occurring with health care groups is the increasing activity in mergers and acquisitions, including the purchase of private practices. Several large health care companies are acquiring health care groups and solo practices to amass health care conglomerates, some now having annual revenues greater then $100 million. Their present concentration seems to be on larger practices (more than 10 providers).

Some organizations place the professional providers on salary. Others

TABLE 5   Comparison of Three Forms of Equity

Characteristic	Sole Proprietor	Partnership	Corporation
Method of creation	Created at will by owner.	Created by agreement of parties.	Charter issued by state.
Legal position	Not a separate entity; owner is the business.	Not a separate legal entity in many states.	Always a legal entity separate and distinct from its owners.
Ownership	Psychologist	Psychologists are general partners; investor is limited partner.	Psychologists and investors.
Capital invested by	Psychologist	Investor	Investor
Liability	Unlimited liability.	Unlimited liability (except for limited partners in a limited partnership).	Limited liability for shareholders.
Duration	Determined by owner; automatically dissolved upon owner's death.	Terminated by agreement of the partners, by the death of one or more partners, by withdrawal of a partner, or by bankruptcy.	Can have perpetual existence.
Transferability of interest	Interest can be transferred, but individual's proprietorship then ends.	Interest can be assigned, but assignee does not have full rights like a partner.	Share of stock can be transferred.
Management	Completely at owner's discretion.	General partners have direct and equal voice unless stated otherwise; limited partner has no management rights.	Shareholders elect directors, who set policy and appoint officers.

Taxation	Owner pays personal taxes on business income.	Each partner pays share of income taxes on net profits, whether or not they are distributed.	Double taxation—corporation pays income tax on net profits, with no deduction for dividends; shareholders pay income tax on disbursed dividends.
Organizational fees, annual license fees, annual reports	None	None	All required.

buy the office, equipment and non-health care assets of the practice and manage the business activities for a fee of about 7% of patient revenue.

INTERNAL SOURCES OF FINANCING

A group of psychologists may also finance their practice internally by retaining earnings rather than distributing cash earned at the end of the year. Cash generated from patient visits has the greatest flexibility for potential use, since the only constraint on using it is the discretion of the practice's owners.

Retained earnings are sometimes difficult to achieve, especially if the practice is organized as a professional partnership, because the psychologist-partners are taxed on their personal tax returns on income the practice retains. If a practice is organized as a professional corporation, it pays corporate taxes on profits. The use of retained earnings as a financing source involves a trade-off of current taxes against the cost of funds if external sources are used.

The direct financing costs of retained earnings are lower than any outside source because there is no interest levied on the funds. There is an opportunity cost, however, since using retained earnings to finance equipment precludes using those monies for any other investment.

SUMMARY

Practices that have planned and budgeted know that sometimes borrowing money is needed to accomplish goals. Debt and equity are the two major categories of financing. Debt incurs an obligation to repay the capital a practice receives. Equity results in transferring a portion of ownership to the lender providing the capital.

Debt financing is available under short-, medium-, and long-term arrangements. A loan's interest rate may be fixed or variable and may be structured with a balloon payment at the end of the loan. Lease financing is a debt instrument that allows a practice to acquire equipment without purchasing it or making a large down payment.

One type of equity financing is the formation of a limited partnership to attract passive investors and provide capital without the practice relinquishing control. A corporation is a legal entity that has an unlimited life and issues stock to raise capital. A joint venture may be formed by several entities to enable a practice to gain access to capital.

3

Lenders

THERE ARE NUMEROUS FINANCING *sources available for psychologists in groups of all sizes. Options range from venture capitalists to life insurance companies, to name only two. Each source of capital has advantages and may be better suited to one's particular financing needs than others.*

This chapter begins by discussing venture capitalists as a source of capital. It then focuses on sources of debt financing, with an overview of banks, leasing companies, thrift institutions, life insurance companies, commercial finance organizations, and venture capitalists. The chapter continues by reviewing the process a practice may undergo in selecting a lending source. Finally, it concludes with a discussion of the evaluation process typically used by lenders.

VENTURE CAPITAL FIRMS

Venture capital firms are generally interested in equity investments in companies with extremely high growth potential and in entities that plan to go public at some time. If a practice's plans include expansion to fill unmet needs in the behavioral health market, venture capital may be a viable option. As compensation for the risk of the practice, venture capitalists may demand a voice in company management and a seat on the board of directors.

Venture capitalists are a diverse group. Targeting the right listing of venture capital companies is an exercise in and of itself. Such companies vary by geographical region, industry specialization, stage of company development, and size of investment preferences. They typically require a comprehensive business plan to serve as a roadmap of a practice's development, financing, operations, and management. For a practice, venture capitalists would focus on some of the following key ideas, which should be communicated in any comprehensive business plan:

- Is the management team for the practice able to grow the business rapidly and successfully?
- Is there a market-driven need for the practice's services?
- Is market potential large enough?
- Do barriers to entry exist?
- How much capital will be required and how will it be utilized?
- What exit strategies are possible?
- Does the practice understand how changes in the local market will affect it?

Practitioners wishing to contact or learn more about venture capital firms are encouraged to write to the National Venture Capital Association at 1655 North Fort Myer Drive, Suite 700, Arlington, VA 22209. The following guides offer additional information on the topic:

- *Pratt's Guide to Venture Capital Sources,* David Schutt and Yong Lim, eds., Venture Economics Publishing, 40 West 57th Street, Suite 802, New York, NY 10019.
- Technology Capital Network, MIT Enterprise Forum of Cambridge, Inc., 201 Vassar Street, Building W59-MIT, Cambridge, MA 02139.

Angels are wealthy individual investors who are former entrepreneurs or executives who act as venture capitalists investing in entrepreneurial companies. Many investment clubs across the country serve as a network to reach this group of investors. The National Venture Capital Association publishes a listing of these clubs.

SOURCES OF DEBT FINANCING

Institutions that provide debt financing include commercial banks, leasing companies, thrift institutions, life insurance companies, and commercial finance companies.

Commercial Banks

Short-term credit from commercial banks is an extremely popular source of financing for all types of businesses, including behavioral health practices. In recent years some banks have set up professional divisions with personal bankers who are experienced in meeting the needs of health care providers.

Bank borrowing may be the least expensive source of debt financing for secured and unsecured working capital loans, equipment loans, and real estate loans. Often, a practice develops a relationship with a local commercial bank and the bank assists in the practice's financial planning process.

Short-term loans offered by commercial banks have several unique characteristics. They are usually extended for a period of 90 days or less and may be secured or unsecured, depending on the amount of risk the bank faces. When a bank loan is secured, the lender normally executes a security agreement in which the practice pledges a certain business asset as collateral. One asset a practice might pledge is its accounts receivable, which are billings to patients and third-party payers for services rendered but not yet paid for. The amount in accounts receivable is an asset that represents money owed to the practice. Additionally, commercial banks may require a personal guarantee by the provider based on personal assets. If the practice does not pledge any collateral against the loan, the bank might extend the loan on the practice's full faith and credit.

Leasing Companies

Leasing has become an increasingly popular source of debt financing. Almost any kind of property can be leased: computer systems, equipment, furniture, and office space. As an alternative to normal debt financing, leasing offers a practice greater flexibility and convenience because the lessor takes on some of the responsibilities of ownership, including maintenance and disposal. If a practice is reluctant to borrow, leasing can be an attractive alternative. The interest rate on a lease will most likely be somewhat higher than a loan extended by a commercial bank because the lessor (i.e., the bank) assumes greater responsibility. Commercial banks and financial services companies are among the institutions that offer lease arrangements.

Thrift Institutions

Thrift institutions—the collective term for savings and loan associations, mutual savings banks, and credit unions—have traditionally been a source of debt financing for borrowers purchasing homes or durable goods.

These organizations were deregulated in 1982 and have become a viable alternative for financing other asset acquisitions, including practices, office buildings, and equipment. Practices seeking debt financing from thrift institutions can expect an environment and terms similar to those of commercial banks. Thrift institutions offer a wide range of services: leasing, credit cards, electronic transfer of funds, and commercial lending.

Life Insurance Companies

Life insurance companies offer limited financing to health care practices in the form of secured real estate loans. Some health care buildings are financed by mortgage loans granted by insurance companies. Low-cost loans are also available from life insurers based on the cash value of a provider's life insurance policies.

Commercial Finance Companies

An alternative source for high-risk borrowers is a commercial finance company, which generally finances credit sales as well as providing funds for short-term purposes. A commercial finance company borrows large sums of money from investors and bankers and then lends it directly to businesses. As a result, its interest rates will almost always be higher than banks, thrift institutions, and life insurance companies, and the terms of the loan reflect the borrower's risky credit rating. Examples of these terms are minimum cash balance requirements; collateral requirements, including personal assets; and remedies for the finance company in the event of default.

Commercial finance companies also provide other services, such as financing and factoring accounts receivable. Since a practice's accounts receivable can be fairly accurately valued and usually easily converted to cash, they are a suitable asset to pledge. As accounts receivable are collected, the indebtedness is reduced. When the full value of the accounts is not pledged, collections made in excess of the borrowed amount are returned to the practice.

In fact, receivables may actually be sold to a financial institution. Commercial finance institutions prefer the sale be made "with recourse," meaning the risk of the account remains with the practice. If accounts receivable are purchased from the practice without recourse, the process is called *factoring*. When a lending institution factors receivables, it assumes the credit risk and the service is more expensive to the practice. Usually, a factor charges a performance commission on invoice amounts and inter-est at 3% to 4% increase over the prime lending rate.

The advantages of receivables financing are that funds can be obtained quickly and there is a more rapid cash flow. Factoring shifts the risk and inconvenience of credit collection to the factor, but both these practices are costly and may make the practice appear to be financially unsound and risky. Selling receivables is not advisable unless the practice is making a large one-time repayment, such as tax bill, or working out a plan to re-cover from a catastrophic event, such as a natural disaster. Providers who sell their receivables to cover monthly operating expenses are borrowing against their own future. It is akin to borrowing against next month's paycheck to pay this month's bills.

SELECTING A LENDER

Even with all the alternative financing sources available, many be-havioral health practices prefer to deal with a bank. No matter who the lender is, it is important to approach the selection by considering the source not only as a current borrowing source but also as one that can supply additional funds at a later date. A practice should select a lender who is responsive, understanding, and committed to the practice's needs. There are three phases involved in selecting an institution:

- Researching potential banking sources
- Interviewing bank officials who will service the account
- Evaluating the candidates

Researching Potential Banking Sources

To determine which bank will best accommodate a practice's needs, it is important to survey local banks and obtain information about their poli-cies and experience in working with health care practices. Sources of in-formation about local banks include other psychologists, other health care providers, other professionals, accountants for the practice, and the attor-ney for the practice.

Once several potential banks have been identified, the practice may contact each one to request financial information, such as annual reports, financial statements, and lending statements. This information should be examined for evidence of financial stability and ability to render services as well as expertise and independence.

- Does the bank have an officer dedicated to health care accounts?
- Has the bank been in the news media recently?
- Are bank officials cooperative about sharing information with the practice?

Table 6 summarizes the typical characteristics of large banks compared to small ones. A practice should use the institution that best meets its needs. Note that the characteristics of individual banks also may vary.

Interviewing Bank Officials

A practice may also arrange for a meeting with bank representatives, especially those who have the authority to guarantee specific services as well as the individual(s) who will be responsible for the practice's account. The practice's expectations and needs from a banking relationship should be discussed, as well as the bank's experience with health care providers.

TABLE 6   Typical Bank Characteristics

Large Banks	Small Banks
More financial resources	Fewer financial resources
Less personal	More personal and involved relationships
More prestigious	More willing to help customers with community and professional introductions
May have professionals who work exclusively with health care providers and other professionals	Interested in customers who add value (professionals)
May have more health care expertise	Many do not have full range of expertise in sophisticated financial instruments
Larger range of total services (executive tax planning, financial planning, investor advice)	May not understand the health care industry
More cautious making loans	May not grow fast enough to continually meet the needs of a growing practice

Obviously, the more familiar a bank is with health care clients, the more likely that it will be able to meet the needs of the practice.

The practice might also query the bank about its staff turnover, especially among senior staff. Having the same personnel over many years will assure their familiarity with the community, the practice, and its operations. Low turnover is also an indication that the bank maintains consistent policies and service offerings. The practice may provide the bank with its brochure or business plan, so that bank officials understand the nature of the practice and what the bank may expect in terms of the practice's needs.

Evaluating the Candidates

The final step in lender selection is evaluating the candidates. The practice compiles and analyzes all the information received from bank interviews and other sources. The bank that offers the best interest rate or the most favorable loan program may not necessarily be the best choice for the practice. The selection should be based on the bank's ability to meet critical banking needs and to provide the services required by the practice. A scenario that might occur is one in which the only bank that will lend the practice money is not the best bank. The practice must then choose to use the bank already willing to loan money. The practice may also change its request or provide additional information and try again with the bank it originally wanted to use.

Qualifications to Look for When Selecting a Bank

- *Competence.* The bank should have experienced, knowledgeable employees who are willing to accommodate the practice.
- *Financial and managerial strength,* including adequate size and stability.
- *Number and quality* of programs geared toward the health care industry, especially experience with behavioral health practices.
- *Competitiveness* of interest rates and loan packages.
- *Willingness to document* the practice's requests in writing as a sign of good faith.
- *Reputation* in the community.

Once a practice has selected a bank, it should consider consolidating all its accounts with that office, including personal, business, savings, and pension accounts. By increasing its business, the practice will increase in importance from the bank's perspective, which may result in preferential treatment for services or more favorable loan terms. Establishing a strong relationship and staying with a bank that provides superior service can be a valuable resource for a practice.

LENDER'S EVALUATION PROCESS

A lender makes a decision about a loan based on its knowledge of the borrower and the practice. A positive impression can be made on a lending officer with a well-prepared and complete set of informational documents. The principal document used to indicate a practice's creditworthiness is its business plan, which is discussed in detail later.

Another key factor that a lender uses in the loan process is its impression of the borrower's credibility. This perception is gained from face-to-face contact between the lender and the practice and with the information provided to support the loan request. Practices borrowing funds for the first time can expect to provide more information to the loan officer than a practice with a credit history with the bank. This information gives the lender a better understanding of the needs of the practice and knowledge about its past credit performance. In order to retain credibility, the practice need only continue to produce results that are consistent with its business plan's objectives and financial projections. A practice that repeatedly returns to its lender for expenses not properly considered in the business plan decreases its chances of receiving favorable terms.

Key Information for Loan Requests

There are three essential items that need to be considered in a loan request:

- How will the money be used?
- How much money is needed?
- How will it be repaid?

Data needed to answer these questions will depend on several things:

- The practice's prior relationship with the bank
- Purpose of the loan
- Amount of the loan

- Percentage of total expenditures being sought (For example, a practice borrowing $5,000 to purchase office furniture valued at $15,000 is borrowing only 33% of the total expenditure, which will be more favorably considered than a loan request of $12,000 for the same purpose.)

Additionally, banks vary with respect to the level of detail they require. For example, if a solo practitioner or group with less than three providers applies for a loan at a local bank, the lender may rely more on personal financial information than on the practice's operating information. On the other hand, if a large practice is financing real estate or a series of capital projects, the institution may require a projected, or pro forma, financial statement showing the capability of the practice's operations and ability to repay the debt. Therefore, it is important to have as much information as possible going into the process.

How the Funds Will Be Used

One major reason a practice might borrow funds is to finance start-up or expansion. When starting or expanding a practice, money is needed to provide working capital, purchase equipment, and pay for office improvements. The lender needs to know how the funds will be used, so that it can obtain a security interest if property and equipment are being acquired. If the funds are to be used for working capital, the bank will require some other form of payment assurance. Also, the purpose of the funds helps determine the interest rate and terms of the loan. For example, the term of a loan to purchase a computer system would probably equal the useful life of the equipment.

How Much Money Is Needed

The size of a loan depends on several factors. First, the total planned expenditure and the amount that will be financed should be determined. This relates to the planning process, as discussed in the first chapter. A practice might invest some of its own funds and borrow only a portion of the total. Next, the expenditure should be included in the business plan developed to support the loan application. This pro forma plan shows the practice's future needs as well as the level of debt it can repay. Finally, the bank must understand how the loan relates to the practice's strategic plan. For example, if a practice is adding providers and needs $100,000 to expand, will that amount be used for working capital and improvements? Will another loan be required for any related issues? A practice may find it is easier to repay excess funds than obtain additional funding if the size of the first loan is insufficient.

How the Loan Will Be Repaid

The practice will be expected to demonstrate to the bank its ability to repay the loan. The main evidence is its business plan, which illustrates the practice's capability to repay the debt from projected income in excess of expenses. The practice may also need a contingency plan showing what steps would be taken if the financial projections proved incorrect. The contingency plan may indicate a source of repayment other than practice income, such as a guarantee based on the personal assets of the providers.

Common Evaluation Criteria Used by Lenders

Bankers consider several factors, known as the six Cs, when evaluating a credit application:

- character
- capital
- capacity
- collateral
- circumstances
- coverage

Character is an intangible and subjective quality that is important to the lender's belief that the borrower will repay the debt. The lender attempts to measure character through analysis of the applicant's credit history; references, including the practice's accountant and the practice's attorney; level of preparation in forecasting ability to repay debt; and the practice's attention to its budget and cash flow. The bank may consider all these factors and make a judgment about the practice. The more familiar the lending officer is with the applicant, the more likely a favorable character judgment.

Capital is the amount of owner's equity in the form of cash the providers have contributed to the practice. A group practice with a large amount of equity indicates a high level of commitment from the psychologists to the future plans of the practice. When the risks associated with a practice increase, banks begin insisting on a greater amount of equity investment by the owner. The larger the equity is, the less the practice needs to borrow and the financial leverage exists.

The proportion of debt to equity may be an important consideration in the overall capital structure. A *debt-to-capitalization ratio* measures the financial leverage of a practice. It is computed by dividing the total debt of the practice by the total debt plus the total owner's equity. Most banks prefer a ratio of 75% or lower. For example, if a practice owes $15,000 and has an additional equity of $10,000 in the practice, the debt-to-capitalization ratio is $15,000/$25,000 or 60%.

Capacity is the practice's ability to use borrowed funds in a prudent and profitable manner. A bank wants to determine if the practice can meet its debt service obligation over the life of the loan. To determine if a practice has capacity, the bank may review the practice's business and marketing plans and judge its ability to sustain its current volume of patients and to attract new ones.

Assets with resale value that are pledged as security for a loan are termed *collateral*. Unless a practice owns the building space it operates in, the marketable assets (those able to be sold) of a practice are basically limited to its equipment and accounts receivable. Both of these assets may be difficult to convert quickly into cash in the event of a loan default, so banks often discount their value heavily. Many behavioral health practices have low levels of collateral; therefore, banks often require that guarantees by the psychologists be offered as a secondary source of funds. Relatives of the psychologists also can make these guarantees.

Circumstances reflect the ability of a practice to generate sufficient revenue to meet its debt service obligations. Circumstances depend on the target market and the demand for services. The criteria used are both current and long-term prospects. The bank appraises, among other things, the ability of patients to pay for the services rendered and the amount and type of competition. The marketing plan may provide adequate documentation to enable the lender to judge whether the practice will be able to meet its obligations.

Coverage refers to the ability to meet debt obligations under unforeseen circumstances. An example would be insurance to protect the practice in the event of the death of a key psychologist or the lack of patient visits in a natural disaster. A *debt service ratio* can be computed to determine the level of coverage by dividing the practice's monthly net income (after compensation, interest, and depreciation expenses) by the proposed monthly payment. The income statement and cash flow statement may

TABLE 7   Loan Application Requirements

Loan Requirements	Reason Banks Ask for Information
Business plan	Overall background; indication of the use of funds in relation to long-range goals
Financial statements (balance sheet, cash flow, and income statement)	Broad perspective of business position, financial strengths and weaknesses
Income tax returns for 3–5 years	Broad perspective of business position, financial strengths and weaknesses
Credit check	Financial solvency
Collateral	Financial safeguard
Cash flow analysis, prior and future years	Assures practice has enough cash to repay the debt
Financial ratios	Business position; ability to repay debt
Evaluation of overall management capabilities	Relationship of management to profitability
Check that practice is legally formed	Safeguard bank against fraudulent loans

be used to show the cash generated by the practice. A practice may also call upon its accountant for assistance in developing the required evidence of coverage. A ratio lower than one indicates the practice is unlikely to produce enough cash to make the payments. Obviously, the higher the ratio, the more confident the lender will feel about extending a loan. For psychologists who are just starting a practice, there may be no prior experience upon which to judge the practice's ability to cover the debt service requirement. In this case, the loan may be restructured to defer initial payments until the practice has an established clientele.

PROCEDURE OF CREDIT ANALYSIS

The procedure a bank uses to analyze a loan application centers on two sets of documentation: the business plan and the financial statements for the practice. Other information such as a personal financial statement may be required to complete the overall assessment of the borrower's creditworthiness. The amount of information required depends on the bank, the practice, and their relationship. Table 7 summarizes most of the items typically required in an application as well as the purpose it serves.

With respect to financial statements, a bank will examine them closely and look for certain relationships that may affect the practice's ability to repay the loan. Specifically, the bank may explore the following:

- **Receivables**
    Amount
    Percentage of past-due accounts
    Average age
    Largest accounts and percentage of total

If the practice has a large amount of receivables or a high percentage of its business revenues in receivables, it may be less likely to be able to repay a loan. The age of a receivable is the length of time between the patient visit and when the bill is paid. As accounts age, the likelihood of the practice getting paid decreases. The largest accounts and percentage of total are important because they show if there are many small receivables outstanding or a few large ones, which may affect the bank's determination of how likely the practice is to ultimately collect the money.

- **Equipment**
    Amount
    List of type, age, and condition
    Appraisal
    Replacement schedule

This information helps the bank determine if the practice will need to purchase or replace equipment soon, thus making it more likely to need another loan. It also shows the bank that the equipment might be worth if the practice were to default on the loan.

- **Loans to other psychologists**

Here, the bank looks at its past experience with other practices and may assume all behavioral health practices will behave similarly.

- **Overextended credit position**

This information tells the bank if the practice is already heavily in debt and therefore more likely to default on a loan.

Indicators of Creditworthiness

Lenders use certain financial ratios to compare the performance of a practice with similar types of borrowers to assess the practice's creditworthiness.

All ratios are evaluated together and in the context of other factors in the financial analysis of the practice's operations and financial position. Table 8 summarizes several commonly used ratios, their computation, the target number that banks expect, and a description of what the ratio measures

Proposal Package

Once a funding plan has been decided (amount of loan, term, interest rate, collateral required, etc.), the formal funding proposal package is completed and submitted to the funding source. Usually, a loan application form is required. A sample loan application is shown as an appendix to this chapter. The proposal package includes the following information:

- Business plan
- Financial statements, including a thorough explanation of any losses or unusual events in the past 3 years
- Budgets and projections, as well as a comparison of actual expenses to budgeted projections for the past year
- Information about providers (e.g., experience, education) or the practice's brochure
- Market value and appraised value of investments and fixed assets (from balance sheet or accountant)

If collateral is required, a clear specification of the pledged items is included in the proposal. If personal guarantees are made, personal financial statements are included as well.

After the practice submits the application and other information, the loan officer evaluates the application, a process that takes 1 to 4 weeks. If the practice has not heard from the institution after 4 to 6 weeks, someone should phone the bank and inquire about the status of the application.

If the lender grants the loan, a preliminary contract or commitment letter is prepared by the lender that spells out the terms of the forthcoming formal loan contract and requires the borrower to sign in agreement to the conditions. The bank may also require a commitment or application fee as a sign of good faith and to offset its administrative costs. The practice may try to negotiate to reduce or eliminate the fee, but the bank may have a policy against it. After the commitment letter has been signed and received by the lender, the formal loan agreement is executed.

TABLE 8 Commonly Used Financial Ratios

Ratio	Computation	Target	What It Measures
Debt service coverage	Net income (after salaries) ± depreciation + interest ÷ (principal + interest payment)	1.5+	Ability of the practice to generate enough cash to repay the loan
Debt to capitalization	Total debt (including lease) ÷ (total debt + equity)	75% or more	Amount of debt the practice has consumed
Return on equity	Net income x 2 ÷ (equity at beginning of year + equity at end of year)	10% or more	Profitability
Current ratio	Current assets ÷ current liabilities	2:1 or more	Ability of the practice to meet short-term requirements
Day cash balance	Cash x 260 ÷ (annual operating expenses)	20 or more	Number of days cash available

The loan agreement may specify certain conditions that the borrower agrees to meet during the life of the loan. Some stipulations include:

- Prevention of additional indebtedness
- Maintenance of a minimum level of working capital
- Restrictions on dividend payments
- Restrictions on mergers or acquisitions
- Limits on capital expenditures within a specified amount
- Limits on loans to officers if the practice is a corporation
- Periodic appraisals of real estate collateral
- Annual audit or review by an independent certified public accountant

The loan's structure becomes a critical issue when the loan is approved. The practice is advised to establish a realistic payment schedule that does not put unreasonable financial burdens on it yet assures prompt, regular payments to the lender.

If the lender rejects the loan application, the practice has a right to an explanation and, if possible, to provide additional data to rebut any negative information. A rejected applicant might successfully apply to another lending institution because different institutions have different criteria and standards and the evaluation of creditworthiness has a substantial element of subjectivity.

MANAGING BANKING RELATIONSHIPS

After a practice has secured the appropriate financing and established the required credit line and checking accounts at a commercial bank, the task of managing its finances does not end. A good relationship with a bank is very important in today's volatile environment and helps ensure that the most appropriate services are received. A practice may achieve the best results through proactive dealings with its banker.

Develop Written Agreements for Services Provided

In addition to periodic meetings, a practice may have a written agreement with a bank for all services provided. Most banks require that their customers sign standard agreements for lockboxes and wire transfers. Since these agreements protect the bank and limit its liability for errors, the practice's attorney may want to review the documents before the practice representative signs them.

A practice may also obtain a service level agreement with the bank that specifies the minimum level of quality of the bank guarantees and, if not met, how much fee discount will be credited.

SUMMARY

Although psychologists often rely on commercial banks for funding, there are other financing sources available, such as leasing companies, thrift institutions, life insurance companies, and commercial finance companies. A practice is advised to select a bank carefully based on which bank best meets its needs. The bank with the lowest interest rate on loans may or may not be the best for a particular practice.

FIGURE 7 Sample loan application.

Application for Loan

Check appropriate box:

Individual - I am applying for individual credit and will rely on my own income and assets to repay any loan (Leave blank the spaces that ask about Applicant #2)

Joint - We are applying for credit together. We want you to look at all our income and assets in evaluating this application. (Complete all sections)

Amount of loan request	Check if	Home purchase/refinance
$		Home improvement
	All other loans indicate purpose	

Applicant #1		Applicant #2	
NAME		NAME	
NO. YEARS AT PRESENT ADDRESS — OWN RENT MO. PAYMENT		NO. YEARS AT PRESENT ADDRESS — OWN RENT MO. PAYMENT	
STREET		STREET	
CITY/STATE/ZIP		CITY/STATE/ZIP	
FORMER ADDRESS IF LESS THAN 2 YEARS AT PRESENT ADDRESS		FORMER ADDRESS IF LESS THAN 2 YEARS AT PRESENT ADDRESS	
CITY/STATE/ZIP		CITY/STATE/ZIP	
YEARS AT FORMER ADDRESS — OWN RENT		YEARS AT FORMER ADDRESS — OWN RENT	
US CITIZEN YES NO	BIRTHDATE MO/DAY/YR	US CITIZEN YES NO	BIRTHDATE MO/DAY/YR
IF COLLATERAL IS OFFERED, PLEASE INDICATE MARITAL STATUS — MARRIED SEPARATED UNMARRIED		IF COLLATERAL IS OFFERED, PLEASE INDICATE MARITAL STATUS — MARRIED SEPARATED UNMARRIED	
NAME AND ADDRESS OF EMPLOYER		NAME AND ADDRESS OF EMPLOYER	
YEARS ON THIS JOB	SELF-EMPLOYED	YEARS ON THIS JOB	SELF-EMPLOYED
GROSS MO. PAY $	NET TAKE HOME $	GROSS MO. PAY $	NET TAKE HOME $
POSITION/TITLE	TYPE OF BUSINESS	POSITION/TITLE	TYPE OF BUSINESS
HOME PHONE	BUSINESS PHONE	HOME PHONE	BUSINESS PHONE

Source of other income (if any)

1 APPLICANT #1	Notice: alimony, child support or separate maintenance income need not be revealed if	MONTHLY AMOUNT
2 APPLICANT #2	an applicant does not choose to have it considered as a basis for repaying the loan	

If employed in current position for less than two years complete the following

1/2	PREVIOUS EMPLOYER/SCHOOL		CITY/STATE		
TYPE OF BUSINESS		POSITION/TITLE		DATES FROM/TO	MONTHLY INCOME

APPLICATION MUST BE FILLED OUT AND SIGNED ON REVERSE

(continued)

Liabilities

Current obligations including banks, finance co., dept. stores and credit cards. Indicate debts of applicant #1 with "1" and debts of applicant #2 as "2". Indicate debts which are jointly obligated as "J".

AUTO YR AND MAKE	FINANCED BY	1/2/J	MONTHLY PAYMENT	BALANCE
AUTO YR AND MAKE	FINANCED BY			
SECOND MORTGAGE TO WHOM PAID	ACCOUNT NUMBER			
OTHER DEBTS-OWED TO				
ARE YOU GUARANTOR OR CO-SIGNER FOR ANYONE?	NO	YES (IF YES, LIST)		

Schedule of real estate owned

LOCATION AND TYPE OF PROPERTY INCLUDING RESIDENCE	TITLED IN NAME 1/2/J	TRUST HOLDER NAME & ACCOUNT NUMBER	DATE ACQUIRED	PURCHASE PRICE	CURRENT MKT VALUE	MO. RENTAL INCOME	MONTHLY PAYMENT	MORTGAGE BALANCE

Miscellaneous information [indicate (1), (2) or (J) as appropriate]

FACE AMT OF LIFE INSURANCE COMPANY _____ _____	BANKING RELATIONSHIPS
	ACCOUNT NO. BALANCE NAME OF BANK
	CHECKING _____
VALUE OF STOCKS AND BONDS	SAVINGS _____

NAME AND ADDRESS OF NEAREST RELATIVE NOT LIVING WITH APPLICANT #1

NAME AND ADDRESS OF NEAREST RELATIVE NOT LIVING WITH APPLICANT #2

HAS EITHER APPLICANT EVER BEEN PARTY TO ANY SUITS, JUDGMENTS, GARNISHMENTS, BANKRUPTCY OR OTHER LEGAL PROCEEDINGS   NO   YES (IF SO, GIVE PARTICULARS)

You may check my credit and employment history and answer any question about your credit experience with me. Everything I have stated in this application is correct and accurate to the best of my knowledge. Under penalty of perjury, I certify that I have provided my correct Social Security Number (Taxpayer Identification Number) and that I am not subject to Internal Revenue Service withholding. Name and Taxpayer Identification Number of applicant #1 will be used for IRS information reporting, if applicable.

_____	_____	_____	_____
APPLICANT #1 SIGNATURE	DATE	APPLICANT #2 SIGNATURE	DATE
_____		_____	
SOCIAL SECURITY NUMBER		SOCIAL SECURITY NUMBER	

4

Preparing a Business Plan

I N THIS TEXT WE HAVE *explored how to determine a practice's financial needs and the types of financing mechanisms that are available. A comprehensive business plan is often a prerequisite to obtaining financing. This chapter begins by defining what a business plan is and when it is recommended for a practice to prepare one. Next, it discusses the various elements of a business plan: statement of objectives, organization, market data, description of services, and financial statements. Finally, it examines the business plan as a practice tool and gives an overview of personal financial statements.*

A well-written business plan is a key determinant in obtaining credit. Planning is a continuing and central activity in every business. The use of a business plan is becoming increasingly more necessary as a tool that enables a practice to obtain financing. A plan is also useful for long-range planning of operations. A business plan accomplishes several items:

- Helps the business obtain financing by gaining the confidence of lenders and investors
- Defines the objectives of the business and builds consensus on how it (i.e., the practice) can reach those objectives
- Allocates scarce resources, especially cash

WHAT IS A BUSINESS PLAN?

A business plan is an organized document that specifies a practice's goals and objectives and projects the overall direction of the practice. It plans the use of resources, market forces, and people skills necessary to meet the stated goals and objectives. It is a blueprint for what is expected to happen in the future and how the practice plans to take control of those areas that can be influenced. In effect, a business plan is a budget written in general terms and serves as a plan of action.

A business plan is two things: a sales document to be used in obtaining financing and an overall operating plan for start-up and ongoing operations. Although the role of a business plan in obtaining financing has been the focus here, its role in practice management is equally important.

The form of businesses varies considerably. Although they may have the same outline, the business plan for a start-up practice would differ substantially from that of an existing practice. For example, a well-established behavioral health practice may concentrate its plan in the financial and cash flow area. A newly formed practice will need to include detailed sections on marketing and operations. In addition, the business plan for a start-up practice is usually more comprehensive and detailed. Business plans for existing businesses, particularly those not seeking outside capital, are usually some adaptation of the original business plan with alterations made by eliminating some initial detail and focusing more directly on financial data.

When Is a Business Plan Recommended?

All practices, regardless of size, should prepare a business plan. There are several occasions when it is particularly recommended for a behavioral health practice to complete one:

- When starting a new practice
- When the practice is uncertain about the level of borrowing it needs
- When multiple financing needs exist
- When requesting large loans (more than can be repaid in a year)
- When requesting loans for start-up capital, working capital, and major practice expansions

A business plan does not need to be specially prepared or presented when a practice is seeking a loan for minor equipment, if the practice can demonstrate a source of repayment for the loan and offer a personal guarantee. The circumstances vary according to the practice, the lender, and their relationship.

Ideally, a practice will have its most qualified person accept responsibility for completing the business plan. However, outside assistance may be found through several sources, including:

- Practice's accountant
- Outside consultant
- Financial planner
- Investment adviser
- College or university small business development center
- Small Business Administration counselor

Each professional will have strengths and weaknesses in completing a business plan, and skill and care will vary by individual. Providers know their practices the best but may not be fully equipped or have the time to write a thorough business plan. A consultant with experience in the behavioral health market can assist in particular areas of the document, including defining the market's dynamics. Thus, an outside professional may only be needed to help prepare a portion of the document. The practice, however, must ensure that the document maintains continuity through each section.

Alternatively, there are several fine off-the-shelf business planning software packages available commercially. Few, if any, are tailored to health care; therefore, some of the sections may not apply to a practice's particular document.

ELEMENTS OF THE BUSINESS PLAN

A typical business plan includes the following items:

- Statement of objectives and action plan
- Description of the organization
- Market data for the relevant area
- Description of planned services and programs
- Financial statements

Statement of Objectives and Action Plan

This section explains a practice's objectives and presents an action plan that integrates all areas of the practice. It describes not only what the practice wants to accomplish but also how it will do so. It includes short- and long-term objectives and answers the following questions:

- Financially, what is the practice trying to accomplish?
- In the course of providing patient care, where will its revenue pri-

marily be generated from—private-pay patients, capitated contracts, other managed care contracts?

- When will the practice accomplish its stated goals and how will it do so?

Refer back to the section on developing goals and objectives in Chapter 1 for further treatment of defining a practice's goals and objectives.

The action plan answers the following questions:

- What are the priorities within the goals and objectives?
- What steps must be taken to meet them?
- Who is responsible for ensuring their successful completion?

The action plan uses the conceptual underpinnings of the goals and objectives to explain how they will be accomplished. It includes dates and priorities. For example, a practice's goals and objectives may state that it wants to have a return on equity of 15%, be a leader in the community, and gain a 10% share of the local market for marriage and family therapy. The action plan prioritizes those items and puts timelines on them. The practice's first priority may be to have a 10% market share in 3 years. To achieve that objective, the practice must have a plan for organizing its marketing effort.

The practice's next priority may be to be a leader in the community, which might be achieved by the provider(s) serving on local boards and conducting educational seminars in conjunction with community leaders in the next 5 years. This objective ties in with the market share objective and may be stated in the marketing plan as well.

Description of Organization

The organization and management section of the business plan includes the following items:

- Brief history of the practice (including where and when it was started)
- Legal form of the practice (partnership, corporation)
- Tax status (S corporation, C corporation, partnership)
- Office location
- Names, credentials, and backgrounds of providers
- Names, credentials, and backgrounds of practice managers (if applicable)

- Achievements and successes of the practice
- Problems or obstacles
- Risks and potential liabilities (include insurance coverage)
- Amount of funding required
- Type of funding required (debt, equity, short-term, etc.)
- How funds will be used
- Current and proposed capital structure (percentage of the practice that is currently funded with debt vs. equity)

Lenders are interested in a practice's clinical capabilities and expertise and its business operations. However, the practice must state how various activities are or will be performed. Coding services, billing, collecting receivables, preparing payroll, and purchasing supplies are all examples of business functions that a well-managed practice must not only perform but perform well.

Marketing Data

This section includes a summary of the geographical area a practice serves and a statement of the practice's marketing objectives and strategy. One reason this is an important section of the business plan is because expected market share is a critical element in determining patient volume. Additionally, pricing considerations affect revenues. This section contains only a cursory discussion of the topic of marketing. For an in-depth review, see the APA Practitioner's Toolbox Series manual *Marketing Your Practice: Creating Opportunities for Success*.

Marketing is the process of identifying what services a practice provides, pricing them, promoting them, and determining how they will be distributed. Generally, marketing involves four steps:

- Analyzing market opportunities
- Selecting target markets
- Developing marketing strategies
- Developing a marketing plan

Analyzing Opportunities in the Local Market

This task starts with a practice assessing its internal environment, external environment, consumers, and competitors. It answers questions as to the relevant internal skills of the practice and the external environment under which is operates:

- Professional skills and areas of expertise within the practice
- Business skills of the practice
- Demographic characteristics of the local area
- Economic climate
- Cultural environment

In addition, the practice attempts to understand the decision-making process of a client when purchasing behavioral health care services. A practice may also identify its consumers and the objectives, strengths, weaknesses, and strategies of its competitors. A practice might consider conducting a patient survey to help gather information.

Selecting Target Markets

The practice then determines the relative attractiveness of entering certain behavioral health services markets by estimating the demand for such services and matching them against the practice's strengths and intentions. The practice next segments the behavioral health services market by classifying patients into groups that behave similarly and then targeting certain segments for the practice's marketing activities. Examples include geriatrics or marriage and family therapy.

Developing Market Strategies

Taking the information about marketing opportunities and target markets, the practice formulates a feasible and coherent marketing strategy that considers the life-cycle (introduction, growth maturity, decline) stage of a particular behavioral health service. In addition, the practice may determine if it wants to be a market leader, setting the pace for the rest of the behavioral health community; a market follower, who lets other practices take the lead; or a niche player, who specializes or concentrates in an area without significantly expanding into the general market.

Developing a Marketing Plan

Making the marketing mix decisions of product, pricing, promotion, and distribution based on the marketing strategies, the practice determines what its office hours need to be, what services it will offer and at what price, and ways it can effectively promote itself, such as through referral sources, educational seminars, and yellow pages ads. The marketing plan may also include a projection of volume by service and payer. This projection may include a start-up period of slowly increasing volume for a new practice.

Description of Planned Services and Programs

This section of the business plan includes a description of the services the practice currently provides now and plans to provide in the future. For many behavioral health practices, this section will be brief but needs to include the following specific items:

- Specialties—What general areas of behavioral health does the practice provide (adolescent, all types, etc.)?
- Tests or specific therapies to be performed—Gives further information on the range of services provided.
- Affiliated health facilities (inpatient facilities, psychiatrists)— Provides the names of facilities where the provider has privileges, the ones customarily used, and providers commonly referred to.
- Provider coverage policies—Who provides emergency and on-call service when the psychologist is unavailable?
- Referral patterns for the continuum of care—Where the patients are often referred from the psychologist.
- Referral sources of patients—Where the provider receives referrals (social workers, judges, etc.).

Projected Financial Statements

The projected financial statements—the balance sheet, income statement, and cash flow statement—are the heart of a business plan. They answer fundamental questions about the practice:

- What is the practice worth today?
- What will it be worth in the future?

If a financial forcecast is prepared properly, it can substantially increase the probability of a practice obtaining capital and can act as a tool to measure the practice's actual performance. If improperly prepared, it can substantially diminish a practice's chances of obtaining financing and increase its risk of not managing itself properly from a financial perspective.

A financial forecast is a practice's best estimate of its most likely results of operations and financial position in the forecast period. A financial forecast needs to be realistic, consider achievable opportunities, and recognize all cost factors and contingencies. This is a conservative and realistic forecast that is used in the business plan for proposals to lenders and investors.

A budget, on the other hand, reflects a practice's planned course of operations during a specific period and is generally structured to motivate performance as well as communicate strategy. A budget may or may not factor in the negative effects of all significant contingencies. In short, a budget is generally more optimistic than a forecast. A budget is prepared as part of the planning process but is not normally an item that is shared outside the practice.

The financial forecast and budget are based on the income statement, cash flow statement, and balance sheet. These three statements are economically linked. A practice cannot attempt to prepare one in the absence of the others. The balance sheet provides a snapshot of a practice's financial picture at one point in time. The income statement provides information about profitability over a period of time but does not provide all the information contained in the cash flow statement. A practice could be operating profitably according to its income statement but have a significant cash flow problem that affects viability.

Developing Assumptions About Financial Statements

A financial forecast is only as good as the assumptions that underlie it. All key assumptions are clearly stated in notes that accompany the financial forecast. Assumptions take into account both internal and external conditions.

External conditions are those that a practice cannot affect, such as:

- Inflation rate
- Behavioral health care market conditions
- Changes in income tax laws
- Changes in health care regulatory requirements
- Changes in coverage policies

Internal conditions are factors that can be influenced by the practice's plans or actions:

- *Revenues*—What are the forecasted revenues by period? What are the revenues by type of service by period (week, month, quarter)? What price changes are reflected in the forecast? What are the revenues by period by major employers, insurers, or others?
- *Costs*—In addition to salaries, what other labor costs are involved in rendering services (pension plans, insurance benefits, etc.)? What other overhead charges (rent, utilities, supplies) exist? What are the marketing costs (advertising, direct mail, visits to referrers)?
- *Accounts receivable*—Forecast the buildup of accounts receivable based on average days bills outstanding and industry receivable turnover statistics. Factor in assumptions regarding discounts, bad debts, and charity care.
- *Capital expenditures*—Forecast capital expenditures based on plans. Forecast major repairs or maintenance items.
- *Financing*—Factor in assumptions about interest rates. Ensure that compensating balance requirements are met in the forecasts. Ensure that target/required financial ratios are met.

None of this is simple. Anyone who has prepared a simple financial forecast or budget by hand knows the frustration of changing even a minor assumption and then redoing the entire forecast. With computer software, however, the drudgery and time consumption of "number crunching" are greatly reduced through the use of electronic spreadsheets or other easy-to-use software applications that make it possible to project the financial impact of forecasted changes in patient encounters, prices, capital expenditures, and other factors to produce a balance sheet, income statement, and cash flow statement using a number of assumptions. Once a practice has developed a basic forecast, it can change the assumptions that affect the financial output and perform "what if" modeling. Providers may consult the APA Practitioner's Toolbox Series manual *Organizing Your Practice Through Automation: Managing Information and Data* for an in-depth discussion of information systems issues.

Using a personal computer, a practice can easily introduce new factors into its projections to determine what would happen if certain events occurred. The process of evaluating the effect of contingencies, commonly described as answering "what if" questions, is a critical part of planning. A complex exercise that otherwise would have required accounting expertise and resources can be simplified to the point where the practitioner or office manager can easily prepare clear and meaningful projections.

The Income Statement

The income statement forecasts a practice's expected results of operation and level of profitability. Generally, lenders like to see a projection period of 1 to 5 years, depending on the size and nature of the loan and the scheduled payback period. Key assumptions that need to be critically reviewed and disclosed in the forecast are as follows.

Services Rendered and Pricing

The number of patient sessions and revenues collected should be estimated realistically in light of the competition and the local market conditions. Investors and lenders sense a danger sign when a practice suggests there is no competition for its services.

Using the number of services rendered (by CPT code) and the price, a practice can determine its projected revenue by multiplying its projected volume by the estimated fees. This amount is then reduced for bad debts, write-offs, and discounts anticipated (the collection ratio).

Expenses

All expense categories should be in the financial forecast. Although some may be subjective, they should be tied to actual forecasts, such as patient encounters or advertising programs. Expenses may include:

- Salaries of psychologists and support staff
- Employee benefits (401K, insurance, etc.)
- Rent
- Utilities
- Supplies
- Leased equipment
- Taxes
- Depreciation expenses

An income statement is shown in Exhibit 6. The Rowan Group is a fictitious practice that is used here as a working example to demonstrate the relationship between the various financial statements.

The Balance Sheet

Balance sheet performance has an impact on cash flow and thus is a key concern to potential lenders and investors. The balance sheet should

Exhibit 6   Income Statement for the Rowan Group

	Jan.	Feb.	Jan. + Feb.	Mar.	Jan., Feb., and Mar.
Revenue	$25,000	$30,000	$55,000	$28,000	$83,000
Expenses					
Support staff salaries	3,000	3,000	6,000	3,000	9,000
Rent	3,000	3,000	6,000	3,000	9,000
Utilities	2,000	2,000	4,000	2,000	6,000
Supplies	500	500	1,000	500	1,500
Telephone	1,000	1,000	2,000	2,000	4,000
Insurance	1,000	1,000	2,000	1,000	3,000
Debt repayment	1,000	1,000	2,000	1,000	3,000
Total	11,500	11,500	23,000	12,500	35,500
Income before psychologist salaries	13,500	18,500	32,000	15,500	47,500
Psychologist salaries	12,000	16,000	30,000	14,000	44,000
Net income	$ 1,500	$ 2,500	$ 2,000	$ 1,500	$ 3,500

be integrated with the assumptions in the income statement and all short- and long-term obligations. A balance sheet statement for the Rowan Group is shown in Exhibit 7.

The Cash Flow Statement

A cash flow statement presents the timing of the receipt and payment of cash flows, including cash generated from patient visits and cash from investments, as well as cash used for operations, capital investments, and debt repayments. The statement also gives information the lender will use to estimate the amount of cash available to cover the planned funding being requested. A cash flow statement for the Rowan Group is shown in Exhibit 8.

Exhit 7   Balance Sheet for the Rowan Group

	Jan. 1, 19XX	Feb. 1, 19XX	Mar. 1, 19XX
Assets			
Cash	$ 57,000	$ 42,000	$ 33,000
Accounts receivable	20,000	35,000	45,000
Supplies	8,000	5,000	9,000
Prepaid insurance	11,000	10,000	9,000
Equipment	125,000	125,000	125,000
Accumulated depreciation	(2,000)	(4,000)	(6,000)
Total	$219,000	$213,000	$215,000
Liability and Equity			
Accounts payable	$ 15,000	$ 6,000	$ 15,000
Interest payable	1,000	2,000	0
Payroll withholdings	3,000	4,000	6,000
Notes payable	100,000	100,000	95,000
Capital stock	0	0	0
Retained earnings	100,000	101,000	99,000
Total	$219,000	$213,000	$215,000

Personal Financial Statements

Frequently, with solo providers and small or new group practices, a lending officer may request information about the personal financial status of the individual provider(s). Providers may be asked to submit statements of their personal net worth, which is a summary of their present financial position. Net worth is defined as a listing of personal assets minus personal liabilities. Examples of each follow:

Assets
- Checking account balances
- Savings account balances
- Certificates of deposit
- U.S. Treasury bills
- Notes receivable (outstanding balance on)
- Stocks (common and preferred)

Exhbit 8   Cash Flow Statement for the Rowan Group

	Month 1	Month 2	Months 1 & 2	Month 3	Months 1, 2, and 3
Operating activities					
Collections for services	$5	$10	$15	$20	$35
Pay various expenses	(15)	(20)	(35)	(15)	(50)
Pay interest	(2)	(2)	(2)	0	(4)
Salary distribution to psychologists	(6)	8	14	(10)	(24)
Cash used by operations	(18)	(4)	(8)	(5)	(43)
Investing Activities					
Purchase equipment	(10)	0	(10)	(5)	(15)
Cash used by investing	(10)	0	(10)	(5)	(15)
Financing Activities					
Invest in practice	75	0	75	0	75
Increase long-term debt	25	0	25	0	25
Reduce long-term debt					
Cash provided (or used) by financing	100	0	100	0	100
Increase (or decrease) in cash	72	(4)	82	(10)	42
Beginning cash balance	0	72	0	82	0
Ending cash balance	$72	$68	$82	$72	$42

- Long-term bonds (corporate, state, U.S.)
- Real estate (at current market value)
- Cash value of life insurance policies
- Automobiles (current market value)
- Other personal property, such as jewelry, furniture, and art (current market value)

Liabilities
- Home mortgage balance
- Automobile loan balance

- Credit card balances
- Other unsecured loans (home improvement, education, etc.)
- Contingent liabilities

A personal financial statement for D. Rowan is given in Exhibit 9.

THE BUSINESS PLAN AS A MANAGEMENT TOOL

With the inclusion of a realistic financial forecast, a business plan guides and helps a practice evaluate its operating results. If, after a practice completes a business plan, it is put in a drawer, so to speak, the practice has missed the point of the process and has thrown away good work as well as a useful tool.

The objectives of the practice should be stated such that plans can be

---

Exhbit 9   Sample Personal Financial Statement

D. Rowan
Personal Financial Statement
As of January 1, 19XX

Assets

Cash in checking account	$ 3,000
Cash in savings account	10,000
Certificates of deposit and money market accounts	50,000
Stocks and bonds	60,000
Cash value of life insurance policy	10,000
Personal automobiles at market value	30,000
Personal home at market value	250,000
Personal assets at market value	45,000
	$458,000

Liabilities

Personal home mortgage balance	$175,000
Automobile loan balance	10,000
Education loan balance	30,000
Credit card balances	5,000
	$220,000
Personal net worth	**$238,000**

measured against actual operating results. The following outline, from another text in this series (APA Practitioner's Toolbox Series manual *Building a Group Practice: Creating a Shared Vision for Success*), can be used as a guideline in developing a business plan for any size practice.

Sample Outline: Business Plan

1. Introduction
    *   Name of the practice.
        *   Form of business entity (i.e., partnership, limited liability corporation, regular corporation, S corporation).
        *   Name and address of primary point of contact for questions regarding the practice's business plan.
        *   One-paragraph summary of the purpose of the enterprise (including a succinct communication of market needs the practice will serve).
        *   If planning a merger, briefly summarize the strengths, weaknesses, profitability, and reason for a good "fit" between the two practices.
        *   Summarize capital requirements.
        *   Discuss the goal of the entity.
        *   What is the group's mission statement?
        *   Briefly, how is success of the organization to be measured?

2. Industry analysis
    *   What factors are motivating this practice?
        *   Discuss industry trends, including managed care, shifting of risk, market consolidation, and development of integrated systems.
        *   What is the industry size and projected growth rate? Discuss nationally and regionally. Be specific in defining market size.
    *   Make reasonable predictions about market trends.
        *   Discuss the impact of recent state and federal legislation and its potential impact on the practice.
        *   Perform a thorough managed care analysis of the *current* market area. Focus on the degree of penetration, payer mix, development of integrated systems, percentages of risk-sharing contracts, requirements for outcome data, etc. Explain how the entity will address these issues.

- Assess the managed care market in 2 to 3 years, if possible. Discuss any relevant trends specific to the local area that may affect decision making.

3. Management Team
   - Organizational chart, if applicable. Show key positions and staff personnel.
     - Identify key management personnel, qualifications (résumés) to manage the entity, experience, and plans to integrate the management and clinical expertise of the practice.
   - Discuss the entitys' compensation plan.
     - Identify the board of directors, executive committee, and trustees, as applicable. Discuss their qualifications, level of authority, and degree of participation in practice dynamics. How will the entity maintain or increase its level of understanding of current behavioral health issues?
     - Identify key supporting expertise, including consultants, lawyers, tax advisers, and accountants.

4. Clinical Services
   - Discuss the practice treatment philosophy.
     - Describe its quality assurance program, including utilization review, case management, clinical protocols, and outcomes measurement.
     - Discuss the contracting strategy. Who does the group contract with? What kinds of payment mechanisms are accepted?
     - Discuss the ability of clinicians (and staff) to operate profitably in a risk-sharing environment.
     - Discuss the importance of customer satisfaction and the use of surveys.
     - Discuss the decision to develop the entity as either a single specialty or multispecialty, substance abuse, or mutidisciplinary group, and how this decision is supported by either financial need or effective market positioning.
     - Discuss the practice's location, building space (lease/purchase), office space, staffing, etc.

5. Marketing Plan
   - Describe and clearly define the entity's market. Discuss geographic size (a map may be helpful here) and potential market growth.

- Identify the customers (patients and payers). Classify market potential according to payer mix and reimbursement methodology (fee-for-service, capitation, etc.). Develop an alternate classification by diagnoses, if possible.
- Discuss strategies to segment and target a specific group in the market. (With fixed resources, namely, time and money, to spend on marketing efforts, where will the practice get the most "bang for the buck"?)
- Include a copy of the marketing plan.
- Who is the competition?
- What is the distinct competitive advantage that differentiates the entity from its competitors (quality, reputation, etc.)? How is this communicated to the target market?
- Discuss the marketing mix, including:

  Company—What are the organization's strengths and weaknesses?

  Customers—Who are they? What do they want in behavioral health services?

  Competition—What are the competitor's strengths and weaknesses? What are the probable courses of action in response to a new entity?

  Price—What is the fee schedule and how is it derived? What is the plan for profitability analysis of capitated contracts? Bundled pricing?

  Location—Where will the main office be located? Are there satellite offices?

  Promotion—How will services be communicated? By what medium and by whom? What will this cost? What is the projected benefit?
- Discuss how the organization will manage customer complaints.

6. Financial Plan (with assistance from a qualified accountant/consultant)
   - Pro forma income statements projected out 3 years.
   - Pro forma balance sheets projected out 3 years.
     - Cash flow analysis, with particular attention to retained earnings, which are especially important when contracting on a risk-sharing basis.

- Break-even analysis, modeled under various assumptions. (Clearly articulate these assumptions.)
- Schedule of capital requirements, including short term (less than 1 year), midterm (years 1–2), and longer term (year 3 and beyond).
- Indicate mechanisms for securing necessary capital.

7. Contingency Planning and Risk Management
- Identify points in the plan that are subject to change.
- Project verbally (and financially) how this will affect the practice.
- Explain the contingency plan(s).

8. Appendixes—Supporting Documents
- Partnership agreements, articles of incorporation.
- Applicable licenses.
- Contracts with other health organizations.
- Insurance policies.
- Marketing materials.
- Résumés.

SUMMARY

A written business plan is often required of a practice requesting a loan. The business plan is a standard way of communicating strategic plans, marketing commitments, financial position, and outlook. The elements of a business plan for a behavioral health practice include a statement of objectives and action plan, a description of the practice, market data, a description of planned services, an income statement, a balance sheet, and a cash flow statement.

Glossary

Access   Patients' ability to obtain needed health services. Measures of access include the location of health facilities and their hours of operation, patient travel time and distance to health facilities, the availability of medical services, and the cost of care.

Acute Care   Health care provided to treat conditions that are short term or episodic in nature.

Ancillary Services   Inpatient hospital services other than bed, board, and nursing care (e.g., drugs, dressings, operating room services, special diets, x-rays, laboratory examinations, anesthesia, medications).

Average Length of Stay (ALOS)   Number of days a patient customarily remains an inpatient for a specified diagnosis or procedure; used in precertification and recertification procedures.

Business Plan   Document that specifies a practice's goals and objectives and projects the overall direction of the practice.

Capital   Financial term for money.

Capitation   Method of payment for health care services in which the provider accepts a fixed amount of payment per subscriber, per period of time, in return for specified services over a specified period of time.

Carrier   Any commercial insurance company.

Carve Out   An arrangement in which coverage for a specific category of services (e.g., mental health/substance abuse, vision care, prescription drugs) is provided through a contract with a separate set of providers. The contract may specify certain payment and utilization management arrangements.

Case Management   Monitoring, planning, and coordination of treatment rendered to patients with conditions that are expected to require high cost or extensive services. Case management is focused and longitudinal, usually following the patient for 3 to 6 months minimum to avoid hospital readmission.

CASE MANAGER   Generic term for various professionals who perform different case management functions, usually working with patients, families, providers, and insurers to coordinate all services deemed necessary to provide a patient with a plan of medically necessary and appropriate health care.

CHAMPUS   (Civilian Health and Medical Program of the Uniformed Services). A health plan of vast size with beneficiaries in all states and a natural field experiment in the use of mental health fee-for-service practices. The patterns of use have major public policy implications for patients' access, provider availability, the cost of alternatives to hospitalization, extent of use, and quality of care.

CLAIMS REVIEW   A review of claims by government, medical foundations, professional review organizations, insurers, or others responsible for payment to determine liability and amount of payment.

COINSURANCE   Cost-sharing ratio between a health plan participant and the insurer or employer. Frequently, the participant is responsible for 20% of covered charges, and the insurer or employer will pay an 80% copayment.

CONCURRENT REVIEW   Third party review of the medical necessity, level of care, length of stay, appropriateness of services, and discharge plan for a patient in a health care facility. Occurs at the time the patient is treated.

CONTINUUM OF CARE   In behavioral health, generally defined as the spectrum of care delivered in residential treatment, inpatient, partial hospitalization, home health, and outpatient settings.

COPAYMENT   Type of cost sharing whereby insured or covered person pays a specified flat fee per unit of service or unit of time (e.g., $10 per office visit, $25 per inpatient hospital day); insurance covers the remainder of the cost.

COST CONTAINMENT   Actions taken by employers and insurers to curtail health care costs (e.g., increasing employee cost sharing, requiring second opinions, preadmission screening).

COST SHARING   Requirement that health care consumers contribute to their own medical care costs through deductibles and coinsurance or copayments.

COVERED EXPENSE (OR COVERED BENEFIT) Health care costs that are specifically cited as reimbursable by the health plan.

CREDENTIALING Process of reviewing a practitioner's credentials (i.e., training, experience, demonstrated ability) for the purpose of determining if criteria for clinical privileges have been met.

DAYS/1,000/YEAR A common measurement used in the health care industry for the ratio of the number of days a patient population has for a particular service per 1,000 members enrolled for a given year. For example, if an HMO with 10,000 members experiences 3,800 total hospital days, the ratio is 380 hospital days per 1,000 members per year.

DAY TREATMENT Intensive care provided on a partial-day basis.

DEBT FINANCING Financing that requires a practice to repay funds it borrows. There is no change in the ownership structure of the practice.

DEDUCTIBLE Flat fee paid by a patient/employee before an insurer assumes liability for all or part of the remaining cost of covered services. Common in major medical policies.

DIAGNOSTIC RELATED GROUPS (DRGs) Reimbursement methodology whereby hospitals receive a fixed fee per patient based on the admitting diagnosis regardless of the length of stay or amount of services received.

DISCHARGE PLANNING Process of identifying, monitoring, counseling, and arranging follow-up care of hospitalized patients. Usually performed by social workers or nurses, the process ensures that patients receive appropriate counseling and follow-up care to assist their convalescence and keep hospital stays at a minimum.

EMPLOYEE ASSISTANCE PROGRAM (EAP) An employer's program of counseling and other forms of assistance for employees experiencing alcoholism or other substance abuse, or emotional/family problems.

ENROLLMENT Means by which a person(s) establishes membership in a group insurance plan.

EQUITY FINANCING Funding that requires the practice to give a portion of practice ownership to the investor providing the funds.

ERISA Employee Retirement Income Security Act of 1974, (P.L. 93-406). Enacted to protect employee pension funds and to encourage the development of other employee benefit plans, including health benefit plans. ERISA has a profound effect on the ability of states to regulate health insurance, employee benefit plans, and related matters.

Excess Charges   Portion of any charge greater than the usual and prevailing charge for a service. A charge is "usual and prevailing" when it does not exceed the typical charge of the provider in the absence of insurance and when it is no greater than the general level of charges for comparable services and supplies made by other providers in the same area.

Exclusive Provider Organization (EPO)   EPOs are similar to PPOs in their organization and purpose; except beneficiaries covered by an EPO are required to receive all of their covered services from providers who participate in the EPO. The EPO does not cover services received from other providers. Some EPOs parallel HMOs in that they not only require exclusive use of the EPO provider network but also use a "gatekeeper" approach to authorize nonprimary care services.

Explanation of Benefits (EOB)   A form provided to a patient (and provider) after a claim has been paid; useful in enabling the patient to check not only benefits received but also the services for which the provider has requested compensation.

Fee for Service   In the traditional fee-for-service model, the provider bills the patient or payer for a specified amount, typically on the basis of the amount of time spent delivering the service. Until recently, providers determined the fees charged for services and customary fees were generally accepted. Now, providers may be required to accept a payer's fee schedule, which demands that a certain fee be accepted as payment in full. PPOs represent an attempt to save the fee-for-service method of payment by regulating the cost of treatment in the context of a traditional reimbursement plan.

Fee Schedule   A listing of accepted fees or predetermined monetary allowances for specified services and procedures.

Fixed Costs   Practice costs, such as salaries and other overhead, that do not change regardless of patient volume.

Free-Standing Facility   Health care center that is physically separated from a hospital or other institution of which it is a legal part or with which it is affiliated, or an independently operated or owned private or public business or enterprise providing limited health care services or range of services, such as ambulatory surgery, hemodialysis treatment, diagnostic tests, or examinations.

GATEKEEPING   Process by which a primary care provider directly provides the primary care to patients and coordinates all diagnostic testing and specialty referrals required for a patient's medical care. Referrals must be preauthorized by the gatekeeper unless there is an emergency. Gatekeeping is a subset of the functions of the primary provider's case manager.

GROUP CONTRACT   An arrangement between a managed care company and the subscribing group that contains rates, performance covenants, relationships among parties, schedule of benefits, and other conditions. The term is generally limited to a 12-month period but may be renewed.

GROUP HEALTH INSURANCE   A single program insuring a group of associated individuals against financial loss resulting from illness or injury.

GROUP MODEL HMO   An HMO that contracts with a primary care or multispecialty group practice for the delivery of health services.

GROUP PRACTICE   A group of practitioners organized as a private partnership, limited liability company, or corporation; participating practitioners share facilities and personnel as well as the earnings from their practice. The providers who make up a practice may represent either a single specialty or a range of specialties.

HEALTH CARE FINANCING ADMINISTRATION (HCFA)   Agency of the U.S. Department of Health and Human Services that is responsible for administering the Medicare program.

HEALTH MAINTENANCE ORGANIZATION (HMO)   A health care delivery system that provides comprehensive health services to an enrolled population frequently for a prepaid fixed (capitated) payment, although other payment arrangements can be made. The organization consists of a network of health care providers rendering a wide range of health services and assumes the financial risks of providing these services. Enrollees generally are not reimbursed for care provided outside the HMO network.

HOLD-HARMLESS CLAUSE   Clause frequently found in managed care contracts whereby an HMO and a provider hold each other not liable for malpractice or corporate malfeasance if either party is found to be liable. Many insurance carriers exclude this type of liability from coverage. It may also refer to language that prohibits a provider from billing a patient whose managed care company becomes insolvent. State and federal regulations may require this language.

INDEMNITY INSURANCE PLAN   An insurance plan that pays specific dollar amounts to an insured individual for specific services and procedures without guaranteeing complete coverage for the full cost of health care services.

INDIVIDUAL PRACTICE ASSOCIATION (IPA) MODEL HMO   An organization that contracts with individual health care professionals to provide services in their own offices for enrollees of a health plan. Specialists are generally paid on a fee-for-service basis, but primary care providers may receive capitated payments.

INTEGRATED CARE   Alternative health care delivery system developed by the American Psychological Association in response to the rising cost of health care services. It is based on six concepts: benefit design, case management and utilization review, communications, direct contracting, network development, and outcomes.

INTEGRATED DELIVERY SYSTEM (IDS)   System of behavioral health care that offers "one-stop shopping" to potential payers, meaning that payers can write one check for the entire delivery of care without having to independently negotiate terms with multiple unconnected providers. IDSs offer a full continuum of care, so patients and premiums are managed within one accountable plan's network of providers.

LEVERAGE   A managed care strategy for controlling costs by steering patients to lower-cost providers called substitutes. In behavioral health care, a clinical social worker's psychiatric nurse may be a substitute for a psychologist.

MANAGED CARE   A means of providing health care services in a defined network of health care providers who are given the responsibility to manage and provide quality, cost-effective care. Increasingly, the term is being used by many analysts to include (in addition to HMOs) PPOs and even forms of indemnity insurance coverage that incorporate preadmission certification and other utilization controls.

MANDATED BENEFITS   Specific treatments, providers, or individuals required by law to be included in commercial health plans.

MARKET SHARE   Percentage of clients served by a practice compared to those counseled by other practices.

MARKETING   Activities structured to communicate a psychologist's skills and willingness to help clients with unmet needs.

MEDICAID   Federally financed state-run health care program for the poor.

MEDICARE   Title XVIII of the Social Security Act. Provides benefits to citizens aged 65 and over and the disabled. Part A covers hospitalization, extended care, and nursing home care; Part B provides medical-surgical benefits.

MENTAL HEALTH AND DRUG ABUSE SERVICES   There are three basic types of mental health services: inpatient care provided in short-term psychiatric units in a general hospital or specialized psychiatric facility; outpatient care for individual or group counseling; and partial hospitalization, a combination of both of the above. See also Employee Assistance Program.

MSO   An entity that usually contracts with practitioner groups, independent practice associations, and medical foundations to provide a range of services required in medical practices, such as accounting, utilization review, and staffing.

MULTISPECIALTY GROUP   Group of doctors who represent various specialties and work together in a group practice.

NETWORK   Group of providers who mutually contract with carriers or employers to provide health care services to participants in a specified managed care plan. A contract determines the payment method and rates, utilization controls, and target utilization rates by plan participants.

NETWORK MODEL   Organizational form in which an HMO contracts for medical services with a network of medical groups. HealthNet, a Blue Cross–sponsored HMO serving Southern California, is an example of a network model. For federal qualification purposes, such models are designated as IPAs.

OPERATIONAL PLANNING   Creation of short-term goals or tactics to achieve long-term goals.

OUT-OF-AREA BENEFITS   Coverage allowed to HMO members for emergency situations outside the HMO's prescribed geographical area.

OUT-OF-AREA CARE   Care received by HMO enrollees when outside the HMO's geographical territory. Services received are usually not pre-arranged by the HMO.

PEER REVIEW   Evaluation by practicing providers (or other qualified professionals) of the quality and efficiency of services ordered or performed by other practicing providers. Medical practices, inpatient hospital and extended care facility analyses, utilization reviews, medical audits, ambulatory care, and claims reviews are all aspects of peer review.

PER DIEM   The negotiated daily rate for delivery of all inpatient hospital services provided in one day regardless of the actual services provided. Per diems can also be developed by the type of care provided (e.g., one per diem rate for adult mental health, a different rate for adolescent substance abuse treatment).

PERFORMANCE STANDARDS   Standards that an individual provider is expected to meet, especially with respect to quality of care. The standards may define the volume of care delivered per a specified time period.

POOL   A large number of small groups or individuals who are analyzed and rated as a single large group for insurance purposes. A risk pool may be any account that attempts to find the claims liability for a group with a common denominator.

PREADMISSION REVIEW   When a provider requests that a patient be hospitalized, another opinion may be sought by the insurer. The second provider reviews the treatment plan, evaluates the patient's condition, and confirms the request for admission or recommends another course of action. Similar to second opinions on surgery.

PREAUTHORIZATION   Review and approval of covered benefits, based on a provider's treatment plan. Some insurers require preauthorization for certain high-cost procedures. Others apply the preauthorization requirement when charges exceed a specified dollar amount.

PRECERTIFICATION   Review of the necessity and length of a recommended hospital stay. Often, certification prior to admission is required for nonemergencies and certification within 48 hours following admission for emergency treatment.

PREEXISTING CONDITION   Any condition for which charges have been incurred during a specified period of time prior to the effective date of an insurance policy. Frequently, a contract with a different insurer will not cover the preexisting conditions of employees or their dependents.

PREFERRED PROVIDER ORGANIZATION (PPO)   Selective contracting agreement with a specified network of health care providers at reduced or negotiated payment rates. In exchange for reduced rates, providers frequently receive expedited claims payments and/or a reasonably predictable market share of patients. Employees may have financial incentives to utilize PPO providers.

PROVIDER   Health care professional (or facility) licensed to provide one or more health care services to patients.

PROVIDER-HOSPITAL ORGANIZATION   Vertically integrated delivery system formed by practitioners and a hospital.

QUALITY ASSURANCE   Activities and programs intended to ensure the quality of care in a defined medical setting or program. Such programs include methods for documenting clinical practice, educational components intended to remedy identified deficiencies in quality, and the components necessary to identify and correct such deficiencies (such as peer or utilization review) and a formal process to assess a program's own effectiveness.

QUALITY MANAGEMENT   A participative intervention in which employees and managers continuously review the quality of the service they provide. The process identifies problems, tests solutions to those problems, and constantly monitors solutions for improvement.

RATING   Process of determining rates or the cost of insurance for individuals, groups, or classes of risk.

RECEIVABLES   Another word for accounts receivable. The amount of money owed a practice for services rendered but not yet collected.

REFERRAL CHANNEL   Generalized category of referral sources. An individual practitioner may be a referral source; family practitioners are a referral channel.

RESIDENTIAL CARE   Care provided in a residential treatment center or group home on a 24-hour-a-day basis.

RISK   The chance or possibility of loss. Risk sharing is often employed as a utilization control mechanism in HMOs. Risk is often defined in insurance terms as the possibility of loss associated with a given population.

RISK POOL   Pool of money used for defined expenses. Commonly, if the money put at risk is not expended by the end of the year, some or all of it is returned to those managing the risk.

SELECTIVE CONTRACTING   Negotiation by third-party payers of a limited number of contracts with health care professionals and facilities in a given service area. Preferential reimbursement practices and/or benefits are then offered to patients seeking care from these providers.

SELF-FUNDING Procedure whereby a firm uses its own funds to pay claims, rather than transferring the financial risks of paying them to an outside insurer in exchange for premium payment. Also referred to as self-insurance. Insurance companies and other third-party administrator organizations may be engaged to process claims or the self-insured company may choose to handle its own. Four forms of claims administration are common:

COST PLUS Third party pays claims and bills the employer for the actual amount of claims in a month (cost) plus an administrative fee to a carrier (plus).

ADMINISTRATIVE SERVICES ONLY (ASO) Employer contracts with a firm to handle claims and make payments for billed services.

SELF-ADMINISTRATION Employer takes on the risk for claims and does the administrative work involved in paying claims.

MINIMUM PREMIUM PLAN Insurance company provides aggregate stop-loss protection plus claims administration services.

STAFF MODEL HMO An HMO in which professional providers in a multi-specialty group are salaried employees of the HMO.

STRATEGIC PLANNING Long-term course of action for a practice to achieve its goals.

STOP-LOSS COVERAGE Insurance for a self-insured plan that reimburses the company for any losses it might incur in its health claims beyond a specified amount.

SUBSTITUTE A provider who replaces another despite differences in training and licensing scope. A clinical social worker and a psychiatric nurse may be substitutes for each other.

THIRD-PARTY ADMINISTRATOR Outside company responsible for handling claims and performing administrative tasks associated with health insurance plan maintenance.

THIRD-PARTY PAYER An organization that pays or insures health care expenses on behalf of beneficiaries or recipients who pay premiums for such coverage.

USUAL, CUSTOMARY, AND REASONABLE (UCR) Charges considered reasonable and that do not exceed those customarily charged for the same service by other providers in the area.

UTILIZATION REVIEW Independent determination of whether health care services are appropriate and medically necessary on a prospective, concurrent, and/or retrospective basis to ensure that appropriate and necessary services are provided. Frequently used to curtail the provision of inappropriate services and/or to ensure that services are provided in the most cost-effective manner.

VALUE-BASED PURCHASING   Selection of a product or service based on criteria other than unit price. Value criteria may include quality, outcome, and access.

VARIABLE COSTS   Practice costs, such as supplies, that change according to the number of patient encounters.

VENTURE CAPITAL FIRMS (OR VENTURE CAPITALISTS)   Firms that provide funding to practices with extremely high growth potential and to those planning to go public.

Bibliography

Brealey, R. A., & Meyers, S. C. (1991). *Principles of Corporate Finance*. New York, NY: McGraw-Hill.

Coopers & Lybrand. (1994). *Growth Company Starter Kit*. New York: Author.

Covert, D. F. (1994). Mercy Medical Foundation of Sacramento: a case study. *Topics in Health Care Financing, 20(2)*, 70–80.

Farber, L. (1994). *Medical Economics Encyclopedia of Practice and Financial Management*. Oradell, NJ: Medical Economics Books.

Hough, D. E. (1995). *Developing a Managed Care Business Plan: A Physician's Guide*. Chicago, IL: American Medical Association.

Manderscheid, R. W. & Sonnenschein, M. A. (1994). *Mental Health, United States 1994*. Rockville, MD: U.S. Department of Health and Human Services.

Pavlock, E. J. (1994). *Financial Management for Medical Groups*. Englewood, CO: Center for Research in Ambulatory Health Care Administration.

DeThomas, A. (1992). *Financing Your Small Business*. Grants Pass, OR: Oasis Press.

Solomon, R. J. (1991). *Clinical Practice Management*. Gaithersburg, MD: Aspen Publishers.

Sterns, J.B., & Johnson, D.M. (1995). Financing alternatives for medical group practices. *Medical Group Management Journal, 45(1)*, 58–62.

Oss, M., & Bengen-Seltzer, M. (1995). Managed care: modern business trends affect behavioral health providers. *Treatment Today, 7(1)*, 48–49.

Starr, B., & Findlay, S. (1994). Mental health: solving the quality problem. *Business & Health, 12(11)*, 23–28.